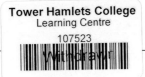

100 Questions & Answers
About Ovarian Cancer

Second Edition

Don S. Dizon, MD, FACP

Assistant Professor OB/Gyn and Medicine
Brown Medical Center
Director of Medical School Program in Women's Oncology
Brown University
Providence, RI

Nadeem R. Abu-Rustum, MD

Associate Attending and Director of Minimally Invasive Surgery
Resident and Medical Student Education Gynecology Service
Department of Surgery
Memorial Sloan-Kettering Cancer Center
New York, NY

Contributors:
Andrea Gibbs Brown, Phyllis Hames,
ZoeAnn King, Marsha P. Posusney

JONES AND BARTLETT PUBLISHERS
Sudbury, Massachusetts
BOSTON   TORONTO   LONDON   SINGAPORE

World Headquarters
Jones and Bartlett Publishers
40 Tall Pine Drive
Sudbury, MA 01776
978-443-5000
info@jbpub.com
www.jbpub.com

Jones and Bartlett Publishers
Canada
6339 Ormindale Way
Mississauga, Ontario L5V 1J2
CANADA

Jones and Bartlett Publishers
International
Barb House, Barb Mews
London W6 7PA
UK

Jones and Bartlett's books and products are available through most bookstores and online booksellers. To contact Jones and Bartlett Publishers directly, call 800-832-0034, fax 978-443-8000, or visit our website, www.jbpub.com.

Substantial discounts on bulk quantities of Jones and Bartlett's publications are available to corporations, professional associations, and other qualified organizations. For details and specific discount information, contact the special sales department at Jones and Bartlett via the above contact information or send an email to specialsales@jbpub.com.

Production Credits

Executive Publisher: Christopher Davis
Editorial Assistant: Kathy Richardson
Production Director: Amy Rose
Marketing Associate: Laura Kavigian
Manufacturing Buyer: Therese Connell
Composition: Appingo

Cover Design: Kate Ternullo
Cover Image: © absolut/ShutterStock, Inc.;
 © Jason Stitt/ShutterStock, Inc.; and
 © Photodisc
Printing and Binding: Malloy, Inc.
Cover Printing: Malloy, Inc.

Library of Congress Cataloging-in-Publication Data
Dizon, Don S.
 100 questions and answers about ovarian cancer / Don S. Dizon, Nadeem R. Abu-Rustum. — 2nd ed.
  p. cm.
 Includes index.
 ISBN-13: 978-0-7637-4311-6
 ISBN-10: 0-7637-4311-9
 1. Ovaries—Cancer—Popular works. I. Abu-Rustum, Nadeem R. II. Title. III. Title: One hundred questions and answers about ovarian cancer.
 RC280.O8D55 2006
 616.99'465—dc22

                    2006023187
6048

The authors, editor, and publisher have made every effort to provide accurate information. However, they are not responsible for errors, omissions, or for any outcomes related to the use of the contents of this book and take no responsibility for the use of the products and procedures described. Treatments and side effects described in this book may not be applicable to all people; likewise, some people may require a dose or experience a side effect that is not described herein. Drugs and medical devices are discussed that may have limited availability controlled by the Food and Drug Administration (FDA) for use only in a research study or clinical trial. Research, clinical practice, and government regulations often change the accepted standard in this field. When consideration is being given to use of any drug in the clinical setting, the health care provider or reader is responsible for determining FDA status of the drug, reading the package insert, and reviewing prescribing information for the most up-to-date recommendations on dose, precautions, and contraindications, and determining the appropriate usage for the product. This is especially important in the case of drugs that are new or seldom used.

Printed in the United States of America
10 09 08 07 06   10 9 8 7 6 5 4 3 2 1

Dedication

The second edition of this book is dedicated in loving memory to Andrea Gibbs Brown.
—Don S. Dizon, MD

In memory of my aunt, Mona Nader, for her kindness throughout her life and her brave fight against ovarian cancer.
—Nadeem R. Abu-Rustum, MD

CONTENTS

When I was diagnosed with ovarian cancer in 1993, the only information available to women like me was statistics about the poor prognosis. Most of us were gripped by the fear of what had happened to Gilda Radner. There was virtually no useful information that helped women understand and learn about the various types of ovarian cancer, treatment options, or how to cope with side effects. Despite the fact that I was unaware that the changes in my body were symptoms of ovarian cancer, I was one of the lucky ones whose cancer was identified early. Women should not have to depend on luck for a cancer diagnosis. This disease truly was "silent." How I wish this excellent book had been available to me and the thousands of other women who were searching for answers to their questions, and most of all, for the realistic hope that the information in this book can inspire.

Receiving a diagnosis of cancer is extremely confusing and emotional. Thanks to the increasing attention that journalists, health and policy leaders, writers, and publishers are beginning to pay to ovarian cancer, more women are becoming aware of this once-called "silent disease." With the recognition that ovarian cancer has begun to receive—and this book exemplifies the best of that attention—women will no longer have to struggle to secure information to make timely decisions. *100 Questions & Answers* will help lead many women into the age of enlightenment about ovarian cancer!

Don't get me wrong—this was not an era that we sought. However, once we find ourselves here, it is essential that we have the knowledge to navigate through the maze of medical terms, distinctions among therapies, and other health issues we never before confronted. This book does just that.

100 Questions & Answers discusses the new therapies, not available to women like me diagnosed 10 years ago, that have helped prolong survival. It also helps the reader understand risks and risk reduction strategies so that healthy women can gain the knowledge that might help them lower their risk of ovarian cancer or catch it in its earliest and most curable stage. With this and other information about symptoms, and the importance of second opinions and surgery by a gynecologic oncologist, this book is essential reading for the general medical community—nurse practitioners, primary care physicians, and obstetricians and gynecologists, who often are the first people to see women with symptoms.

Finally, this important book provides useful references to other books, articles, Web sites and support groups, and advocacy organizations, such as the Ovarian Cancer National Alliance. Together they offer women and their families educational materials, the latest information about treatment options, community resources, and opportunities to raise awareness about this disease.

In fact, just as resources like this book have dramatically changed how women approach their battles with ovarian cancer, so too has the advent of a national advocacy movement that joins survivors, family members, and medical professionals in a united effort to conquer this disease. Like most movements, the ovarian cancer movement began at the community level and was led by women who were determined to make ovarian cancer "silent no more." The movement got a big boost when several of these women gathered in Indianapolis in the spring of 1997 and determined that there was a need for "something more." And thus was born the Ovarian Cancer National Alliance—a national umbrella organization that unites the efforts of individuals and groups across the country to focus national attention on ovarian cancer. Because there is not a reliable screening tool for ovarian cancer, the Alliance has kept its main focus on public education. "Until there's a test, Awareness is best!" is our mantra!

Guided by a strong passion to raise awareness about the symptoms and risks of ovarian cancer, to fight for more research funds, to make sure women with ovarian cancer get to the proper specialists and receive optimal treatments, the ovarian cancer community has expanded in many communities across the country and given voice to this once "silent disease." Since the Alliance's founding, these national and local efforts have fueled a dramatic increase in research funds, expanded treatment options, and even improved survival for women battling ovarian cancer.

Heartening, yes. But the Alliance and our supporters are far from satisfied. We urgently need a reliable, easily administered early detection tool. And we will continue to advocate for expanded research funds and more clinical trials so that the next edition of this fine book will include even more answers for women with ovarian cancer.

Patricia A. Goldman
President, Ovarian Cancer National Alliance
July 25, 2003

Ovarian cancer. Two words that can bring a woman's world to a complete standstill. This diagnosis, shared by approximately 20,000 women in the United States each year, is the eighth most common cancer in women, with a lifetime risk of approximately 1% in the general population. Yet we don't know all that much about ovarian cancer. It is not discussed as prominently in the media as other types of cancer, and unless we or someone close to us are diagnosed, we tend not to think much about it.

But the diagnosis can be devastating. Patients and loved ones are overwhelmed by fear and anxiety, confusion, sadness, information overload, and many, many questions. We wonder: What causes ovarian cancer? What are my treatment options? How will treatment affect my body and my mind? Will I have pain? Why did I get this disease? What are the implications for my children and grandchildren? Many questions, and many possible answers. This book is an attempt to answer some of these questions.

Two oncologists with significant input from ovarian cancer patients have worked together to compile information about ovarian cancer that is relevant to the patient and her loved ones. In this second edition we tried to update some of the commonly asked 100 questions and provide some answers relating to new treatments and current options. It is the hope of the authors that the information contained in this book will aid in alleviating some of the uncertainty and confusion felt by many patients and their families who are overwhelmed with information during their diagnosis and subsequent treatment.

Many advances in the treatment of ovarian cancer have been made in recent years, both from the surgical and medical standpoints, and new clinical trials are ongoing to help discover the most effective and least toxic treatment strategies. We have also made progress in reducing the risk of ovarian cancer in women who may be at increased risk for developing this disease by offering risk-reducing surgery. Hopefully, with continued research and medical advancements, we will be able to find a means to prevent this disease and cure the majority of patients affected by it.

Nadeem R. Abu-Rustum, MD
April 2006

I can honestly say that one of the biggest accomplishments in my life was writing the first edition of *100 Questions & Answers About Ovarian Cancer*. The opportunity to collaborate with Andrea and Nadeem was a fulfilling experience, and it brought forth a bond among three people dedicated to the fight against ovarian cancer, albeit in three different roles.

So much has happened since the book was first published. I made the move from New York City to Providence, Rhode Island, to assume the role of Director of Medical Oncology for the Program in Women's Oncology at Women & Infants' Hospital of Rhode Island. Although I thought I would never see my own patients from Memorial Sloan-Kettering again, I was surprised when after being at this new job for six months, I received a call from Andrea. It turned out that her cancer had recurred as I was leaving New York, and since then, she had been on continuous treatment. Recently, the treatments were less effective and she was once more having disease progression. She was having more symptoms of her cancer, but was still able to maintain her level of activity, though she was no longer working. She wanted to talk about her cancer, and had called to ask if I would resume her care if she decided to come home to Providence, where her parents still lived. "Of course I would," I told her.

When Andrea came to my office, I was so happy to see her. Though much had changed—she was thinner and frailer—her eyes remained vibrant and full of life, and we fell back into a level of comfort more like friends reconnecting than doctor and patient. After reviewing her most recent notes and films, Andrea and I had a long discussion about her disease and the prognosis she faced. We talked about further treatment, side effects of the options left, and her goals. More than living longer, she wanted to live well. She did not want pain, and she did not want to suffer through toxic treatments knowing she could not be cured.

She eventually did move up to Rhode Island to be closer to her family. We chose not to pursue further treatment and instead concentrated on quality of life. Andrea ultimately succumbed to ovarian cancer in October 2004.

Ovarian cancer continues to be a very scary disease, and many women diagnosed feel it is a death sentence. Although Andrea ultimately succumbed to it, it never stopped her while she was alive, and she lived well and lived strong with the disease for five years. Although I lost a good friend, I also keep her memory alive as an inspiration that the fight goes on.

In this second edition, Nadeem and I have revisited the questions, incorporating new ones that have been suggested by readers. We also sought to update existing questions with new information that has come to light since our first publication. Information about the appropriateness of surgery in recurrent disease and the role of intraperitoneal therapy in advanced disease have been included to highlight these gains. We have invited more women to participate with this edition to help provide a multi-person view of this illness, and I am eternally grateful for the contributions of three incredible women, all ovarian cancer survivors: Phyllis Hames, ZoeAnn King, and Marsha Posusney. We also decided to keep some of Andrea's answers to questions, which as I read them once more, ring as true now as they did the first time.

For those with ovarian cancer, and their families, friends, significant others, and loved ones, I hope this book will serve as a resource on practical questions regarding the disease. Those of us who treat ovarian cancer like to think we are doing more than performing surgery or administering chemotherapy or radiation. Every day, women welcome me into their lives and, in the process, I get to know them and their families. It is much more than just treatment; it is a relationship that we all hope will extend through the years. The fact is: We can cure ovarian cancer, but even when we cannot, we can help you live with it, too.

I would like to thank my own family for their constant support, including Henry W. Stoll; our daughter Isabelle; my parents, Millionita and Modesto M. Dizon; my mother-in-law, Marilyn Z. Stoll; and my four sisters, Michelle, Maerica, Precy, and Marie. I would also like to acknowledge the support of my "new" family at Brown in the Program in Women's Oncology: C.O. "Skip" Granai, Paul DiSilvestro, Christina Bandera, Trevor Tejada-Berges, Laurent Brard, Mary Gordinier, Richard Moore, AnnMarie Bradley, Amanda Goldstein, and Nicole Charbonneau, and the staff at the Program in Women's Oncology.

This book is dedicated in loving memory to Andrea Gibbs Brown: Her fight was heroic, her life an inspiration, and her death a constant reminder of all that has yet to be done.

Don S. Dizon, MD, FACP
March 2006

PART ONE

The Basics

Where are my ovaries? What do they do?

What does it mean to have cancer?

What is a cyst? Is it related to ovarian cancer? How do a complex ovarian cyst and a simple cyst differ?

More...

1. Where are my ovaries? What do they do?

An understanding of basic female anatomy and the function of the ovaries is a good starting point for the following discussion of ovarian cancer.

The ovaries, fallopian tubes, and uterus are what make up a woman's internal female reproductive organs (**Figure 1**). These organs lie deep in the pelvis and are connected to one another. The cervix is the external extension of the uterus and, together with the vagina and vulva, forms the female external genital tract.

Each woman is born with two ovaries, located on either side of the pelvis and flanking the uterus. Other organs are located near your ovaries: the small bowel and the **omentum**; the bladder, which sits on top of the uterus; and the rectum, which lies under the uterus.

The ovaries are where eggs are stored. The ovaries start to release eggs when girls reach adolescence, and their bodies prepare themselves for possible pregnancy by the release of

Omentum

Fatty apron that drapes from the stomach and colon.

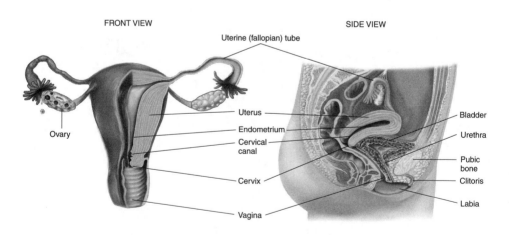

FRONT VIEW   SIDE VIEW

Uterine (fallopian) tube

Ovary

Uterus
Endometrium
Cervical canal

Cervix

Vagina

Bladder
Urethra
Pubic bone
Clitoris
Labia

Figure 1   Anatomy of the female reproductive system. Reproduced from Alters S, *Biology: Understanding Life, Third Edition*. © 1999 Jones and Bartlett Publishers, Inc., Sudbury, MA.

hormones called **estrogen** and progesterone. Eggs are released at monthly intervals (called **ovulation**), and their release begins the menstrual cycle.

The ovaries are essential as the home to those eggs until they're released into the fallopian tube and travel to the uterus. If an egg is not fertilized, the uterus sheds its lining. This process is manifest as menstruation, or your period. The ovaries not only carry a woman's eggs, but also are responsible for the release of estrogen which causes breast development and other sexual characteristics in women.

As a woman ages, the ovaries slowly stop producing hormones, which results in **menopause**. During menopause, the process of egg release slows down and eventually stops. In addition, estrogen production also slows. The uterus responds to changes in hormone levels and doesn't build up as much tissue as it used to, causing periods to become irregular until they, too, eventually stop. The symptoms of menopause occur owing to the gradual decline in the levels of estrogen produced by the ovaries.

Estrogen

A female hormone produced by the ovaries; it is responsible for female changes during maturity.

Ovulation

Process of egg release from the ovary.

Menopause

Physical changes marking the end of a woman's fertile years, the most notable change being the cessation of menstrual cycles.

2. What does it mean to have cancer?

As they do with other organs, a number of diseases and malfunctions can affect the ovaries. Cancer is just one of these. As we get into the discussion of ovarian cancer, we'll describe some common diseases that can be associated with, or sometimes confused with, ovarian cancer, such as ovarian cysts and borderline **tumors** (see Questions 3 and 4). First, however, it is most important that you understand what cancer is—and what it is not.

Tumor

A mass of cells that grow abnormally.

What Cancer Is

Cancer results when a cell starts to grow out of control. Normally, cells follow the same cycle of growth, cell division, and eventual death. When we were still developing, first as babies inside our mothers and continuing on while we were infants

Cancer results when a cell starts to grow out of control.

and children, our cells rapidly grew and divided. The end result was **differentiation**—it's what enabled a red blood cell to carry oxygen, an intestinal cell to absorb food, and an ovary cell to produce hormones to make eggs. If cells are injured or get too old, they undergo a process called **apoptosis**, or programmed cell death. This is what keeps us healthy and all our organs operating normally.

Differentiation

The process of cells maturing so they can perform specific processes in our bodies.

Apoptosis

Programmed cell death.

Some of our organs keep the ability to divide in order to replace dead and dying cells. These include the skin, gastro-intestinal tract, hair follicles, and to a large degree, the ovaries, which replace their surface after an egg is released.

If a cell undergoes changes in its building blocks, called DNA, it can escape this tightly regulated life cycle. These DNA changes, also called mutations, can allow cells to keep growing and dividing. They no longer respond to your body's signals to stop dividing, and this process of unchecked cell division results in a mass of such cells, called a tumor. If a tumor cell breaks free from its origin (in this case, the ovarian cell within the ovary) it can travel through the bloodstream and land in another area of one's body far away (in the lung, for example) and start growing there; it is by definition **metastatic**. These two features—unchecked cell growth and the ability to metastasize—define cancer.

Metastatic

Adjective used to describe a tumor that has spread.

What Cancer Isn't

It's important to state at this point that cancer is not something that can be passed from one person to another, like a virus or bacteria; cancer is not an infectious disease. You can't get cancer from another person, nor can you give it to someone else by simply coming into contact with that person, even close contact. A lot of factors contribute to the development of cancer, and having a family history of cancer is one of them. However, even if your mother had ovarian cancer, it doesn't mean that you will certainly also develop cancer—although you might have a higher risk of getting it than someone whose

Cancer is not an automatic death sentence.

mother did not have it. Most important, cancer is not an automatic death sentence. That's a reaction many people have because, for decades, we lacked effective treatments for most kinds of cancers, and significant fear and stigma were attached to cancer. Thankfully, medicine has come a long way, and although cancer is still a fearsome thing, many people survive it, and some are completely cured. Innovations in treatment and new drugs are developed continually, so that even the most dangerous forms of cancer are becoming increasingly curable as new information about how cancer works is uncovered.

How Cancer Spreads

Cancer can spread in three ways: by extending into surrounding tissue; by passing through the blood supply, a process called hematogenous dissemination; or by traveling in the **lymphatic system**, the "cleaning system" of the body, in a process termed **lymphatic spread**. Knowing the ways in which cancers spread is important, because such knowledge is often used to decide what type of surgery is necessary and what other types of treatment are necessary (such as the use of chemotherapy and the number of cycles needed).

In the case of ovarian cancer, cells that line the ovary acquire genetic mutations that enable them to become cancer. Unlike many other cancers that tend to spread throughout the body, ovarian cancer prefers the environment within the abdominal cavity (also termed the **peritoneum**). Although it can spread to the liver and lungs or to other places, ovarian cancer is more commonly found growing within the pelvis or, when more advanced, in the abdomen. There, it can land anywhere around the abdominal cavity, surrounding the small bowel or **colon**, as a process called **peritoneal seeding** or **carcinomatosis**. These features are used in the staging (or classification) system for ovarian cancer (discussed in Question 17).

Lymphatic system

A network of lymphatic channels, lymph nodes, and organs, such as the spleen and the tonsils, that forms the major component of the immune system.

Lymphatic spread

Metastasis of cancer cells through the lymphatic system.

Peritoneum

The lining of the peritoneal cavity.

Colon

The large intestine, part of your gastrointestinal tract. Its function is to absorb water and food and to excrete stool.

Peritoneal seeding

The process of cancer spreading to involve the peritoneal surface.

Carcinomatosis

Cancer deposits along the abdomen, often along the bowel and involving the omentum.

Computed tomography

Otherwise known as a CT scan, this is a highly sensitive radiology exam used to help diagnose and follow patients with cancer.

Septations

Thin membranes or walls dividing an area into multiple chambers. Often used to describe complex cysts seen on ultrasound.

Anechoic

Used in ultrasound studies, describes a lack of different ultrasound signals, commonly seen with simple cysts.

Multi-compartmental

Multiple spaces, used to describe a finding seen in complex cysts on imaging studies, like ultrasounds.

Echogenic

An ultrasound term describing complex patterns seen within a cyst.

Papilla

Budding formations on structures, seen on ultrasound or other imaging.

3. What is a cyst? Is it related to ovarian cancer? How do a complex ovarian cyst and a simple cyst differ?

A cyst is defined as a fluid-filled growth. Most cysts are not cancer and will go away if left on their own. Ovarian cysts are very common in women before menopause; however, they can also be seen after menopause. On the basis of how they look under ultrasound, **computed tomography (CT)**, or magnetic resonance imaging (MRI), cysts can be one of two types: simple ovarian cysts or complex ovarian cysts.

Simple ovarian cysts are generally thin-walled and contain fluid. As seen on ultrasound, they have a characteristic appearance: They're bland, with a uniform wall around them; they do not have walls within them (also called **septations**); and they do not have differences in their internal appearance (also called **anechoic**). They're common and occur during egg formation, or ovulation.

When an egg forms, it forms in a follicle. If this follicle becomes big enough, it can be seen by ultrasound as a cyst (**Figure 2**); in this situation, they are often termed functional cysts. Cysts appearing this way are generally not cancerous.

Complex ovarian cysts are defined by the presence of internal walls within the cyst (septations) leading to the appearance of different rooms within the cyst (**multicompartmental**), different appearances within the cyst (**echogenic**), the appearance of buds in the cyst cavity (**papilla**), or differences in the thickness of the surrounding wall (**Figure 3**). Complex ovarian cyst walls may be thicker; they may show nodularity, a solid component, or debris. Complex cysts are more of a concern. They may be associated with cancer, particularly after menopause. Additionally, with special ultrasound imaging to assess blood flow (called Doppler imaging), these complex cysts may be found to be vascular, which may also raise concerns about the possibility of cancer.

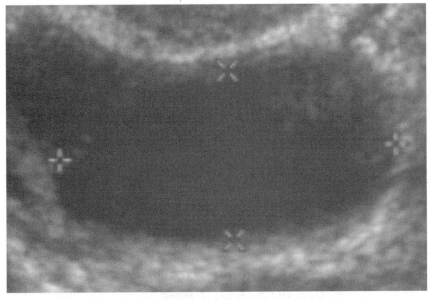

Figure 2   Ultrasound image of a single ovarian cyst.

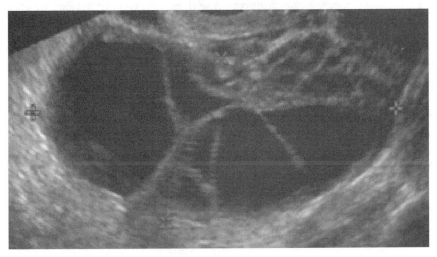

Figure 3   Ultrasound image of a complex ovarian cyst.

The features of the cyst can best be determined by imaging studies, such as a pelvic ultrasound or a pelvic MRI. Depending on the features of the cyst as seen by imaging studies and on other clinical factors, a surgeon will make a decision with a patient as to whether to observe this cyst or to remove it surgically. Observation is commonly used in premenopausal women who have simple cysts or complex cysts that appear to be caused by hemorrhage or bleeding in the ovary, a common occurrence with ovulation.

Surgery is usually considered for large simple cysts that may cause symptoms of pain; for complex cysts with any of the previously discussed findings (papilla, multicompartmental, or thick-walled) at any age; or for complex cysts after menopause. Obtaining a blood tumor marker level, such as that obtained by CA-125 (see Question 15) may be helpful, but the test cannot specifically identify ovarian cancer.

4. What is a tumor? How do benign and malignant tumors differ?

You can develop tumors that aren't cancerous, termed benign.

A tumor is a mass of abnormal cells. To be specific, the term *tumor* is not synonymous with cancer. You can develop tumors that aren't cancerous, termed **benign**. The main difference between a benign tumor and a malignant tumor is that benign tumors do not spread.

Benign
Not cancerous.

In fact, most epithelial ovarian tumors are benign. Examples of these are **adenomas**. However, if a tumor can spread and invade, it is no longer benign and is considered to be malignant. A malignant tumor is synonymous with cancer. Pathologists refer to malignant tumors as carcinomas. The malignant counterparts to the previously mentioned adenomas are **adenocarcinomas**, which are the most common type of ovarian cancer.

Adenomas
Noncancerous tumors arising from epithelial cells.

Adenocarcinomas
Type of cancer, arising from the cells of epithelial origin.

5. What is a borderline tumor? Is it ovarian cancer, or isn't it?

Some women go to their doctor with signs and symptoms of ovarian cancer, undergo surgery to remove the cancer, and then are told, "Don't worry about it; it wasn't cancer after all, it was a borderline tumor." This often results in more confusion and questions than even before the surgery.

Borderline tumors of the ovary do not appear normal through the microscope but do not have the appearance of cancer, either. They show evidence of increased growth and changes in their architecture that may not be considered normal to a pathologist. However, they differ from ovarian cancer because they do not show evidence of invasion into the surrounding ovarian tissue. Therefore, they're placed in an intermediate-risk group of tumors, which is why they're called borderline or are said to have low malignant potential. They are not, strictly speaking, ovarian cancer, but they're nevertheless an abnormality in the ovaries that can be harmful and must be treated.

Borderline tumors account for approximately 15% of all ovarian tumors. They require surgical staging just as ovarian cancers do. Although, by their very definition, they are not invasive, they do have the potential to deposit throughout the abdominal cavity, which is why they require **surgical staging**. In fact, their stage (see Question 17 on page 23 and **Table 4** on page 24) appears to be an important predictor of survival and recurrence.

Stage I patients are likely to be cured at surgery, whereas those with more advanced disease are at greater risk of recurrence. Still, the prognosis of women with borderline tumors is quite good, with more than 85% of patients alive 5 years after diagnosis.

6. What is a dermoid cyst?

A dermoid cyst is the more common name of a mature teratoma, which is a specific type of germ-cell tumor (discussed in Question 8). Dermoid cysts are the most common type of tumor in young women and commonly present as an ovarian mass. They arise when a cell destined to become an egg starts

Borderline

A term used to describe a tumor that does not appear normal but does not meet a pathologist's criteria for cancer; otherwise described as low malignant potential.

Surgical staging

Procedure of determining the extent of cancer present.

to divide within your ovary, rather than dividing and growing in your uterus after it's fertilized. In the process of developing, such cells may also grow into different tissue types, such as teeth, hair, and even lung tissue. Cancer arising from a dermoid cyst is very rare, especially if it occurs in women below the age of 40, and surgery to remove the mass is all that's usually needed. Most women can expect to be cured after surgical removal of this tumor.

7. What is a Krukenberg tumor?

Krukenberg tumor

A cancer that has gone into the ovary from another place, usually starting in the stomach.

Because these tumors arise from somewhere other than the ovary, Krukenberg tumors technically are not ovarian cancer.

It might be confusing to be told that you have a cancerous growth in your ovaries, but you don't have ovarian cancer. The reason for this strange fact is that a type of cancer is always defined by where it started, not where it's found, which means that lung cancer found in the bones is still lung cancer, and breast cancer found in the liver is still breast cancer. This is important because different forms of cancer are treated with different methods: Chemotherapy drugs that work against lung cancer, for instance, may not work as well against breast cancer or ovarian cancer, and vice versa. A **Krukenberg tumor** is cancer that's found in the ovary but started in the gastrointestinal tract, typically in the stomach. Because these tumors arise from somewhere other than the ovary, Krukenberg tumors technically are not ovarian cancer; this term is reserved for cancer that begins in the ovary. Treatment of a Krukenberg tumor is dictated by where it came from originally, so the treatments described in this book probably do not apply to patients with Krukenberg tumors. True ovarian cancer is described in the next section (Question 8).

PART TWO

Risk Factors, Diagnosis, and Staging of Ovarian Cancer

What does it mean to have ovarian cancer?

Are there risk factors for ovarian cancer?

Is hormone replacement therapy associated with ovarian cancer?

More...

8. What does it mean to have ovarian cancer?

Along with the uterus and fallopian tubes, the ovaries comprise the internal female gynecological tract. As discussed in Question 1, the ovaries have two main functions: (1) the release of hormones that regulate menstruation and pregnancy and (2) the storage of eggs. Every time an egg is released, the ovary must repair itself and undergoes a process called **regeneration**, in which the surface is rebuilt.

Regeneration

To grow back.

The ovary is composed of three different cell types, or histology: surface or epithelial tissue; germ cells, which produce eggs; and stromal tissue, the mesh that supports the ovary. All three tissue types can give rise to ovarian cancer, but not all such cancers are treated the same way. This book focuses primarily on the treatment of the epithelial ovarian cancers, unless otherwise stated. **Table 1** lists the types of nonepithelial ovarian cancer.

Table 1 Nonepithelial ovarian cancer

Histology	Percentage of All Ovarian Tumors
Metastatic	5–6%
Sex cord/stromal	5–8%
Germ-cell tumors	3%
Mixed mesodermal tumors	< 1%
Lymphoma	< 1%

Other types of ovarian cancer can occur beyond these, but they're much rarer. These types include **mixed mesodermal tumors** (or carcinosarcomas) and small-cell cancers. The different types of cancer underscore the importance of tissue analysis by a pathologist.

Mixed mesodermal tumors

Tumors of dual origin with one part consisting of carcinomas and the other part consisting of sarcoma, hence their other designation as a carcinosarcoma.

Epithelial ovarian cancer is the most common type of ovarian cancer. It is a cancer that occurs in the surface (epithelium) of the ovaries and, as discussed in Question 9, is related to the frequency of ovulation. Although women of any age can develop it, most commonly it's diagnosed in women older than 60. Estimates claim that more than 25,000 women each year will be diagnosed with this cancer. Epithelial ovarian cancers can be classified further on the basis of the type of cells seen through a microscope. They are serous (most common), mucinous, endometrioid, transitional-cell, and clear-cell types of epithelial ovarian cancers. If a cancer bears no resemblance to any of these types of cancers, is it termed **undifferentiated**. The type of epithelial cancer generally does not alter the treatment plan, although clear-cell cancer may not respond as well as the others to chemotherapy.

Germ-cell tumors arise from the cells that produce eggs. Most germ-cell tumors are diagnosed in young women and make up 20% of all ovarian tumors, of which 3% are malignant. In 90% of cases, they involve only one ovary. Given that these tumors tend to appear in young women who may want to have children at some time, sparing the unaffected ovary is a high priority.

Table 2 lists the different types of germ-cell tumors. The most common type of germ-cell tumor is the dysgerminoma, which represents 50% of all germ-cell tumors. The second most common is the **endodermal sinus**, or yolk-sac tumor. The immature teratoma is the third most common, and prognosis with these is highly dependent on what they look like under the microscope; they are graded as low or high grade by a pathologist, based on the amount of early nerve tissue seen in the tumor itself. Approximately 10% of germ-cell tumors will be made up of various types of tissue and are called mixed germ-cell tumors.

The type of germ-cell tumor that the pathologist finds under the microscope is a crucial factor in determining whether chemotherapy is used after surgery. Women who have had a thorough surgical evaluation and are found to have stage I dysgerminoma or a low-grade immature teratoma do not require chemotherapy and have an excellent **prognosis**.

Undifferentiated

A pathologist's term to describe cellular changes of a cancer cell; this describes cells that bear no resemblance at all to normal cells.

Endodermal sinus tumor

A type of germ-cell tumor, derived from early cells destined to become eggs. Otherwise, they are referred to as yolk-sac tumors.

Prognosis

An estimate of the outlook following the diagnosis of a disease such as cancer.

Table 2   Germ-cell tumors

Dysgerminoma
Endodermal sinus tumor (or yolk-sac tumor)
Embryonal carcinoma
Polyembryoma
Choriocarcinoma

Teratoma
   Mature
   Immature

Mixed germ-cell tumor

A lot of work has been done to identify what factors influence prognosis (prospect for recovery) in women with germ-cell tumors. A poor prognosis is associated with mixed-cell-type tumors, with large tumors (greater than 10 centimeters) that are made up of endodermal sinus tumor, with choriocarcinoma, or with immature teratoma. Tumors measuring less than 10 centimeters were found to offer a good prognosis, regardless of cell type.

Ovarian cancers that arise from the surrounding connective tissue of the ovary are called sex cord–stromal tumors. The cells that give rise to these tumors are responsible for the release of female hormones: estrogen (in the case of Sertoli cell, granulosa cell, and theca cell tumors) and progesterone (in the case of Sertoli-Leydig and steroid cell tumors). Sex cord–stromal tumors account for 5% of all ovarian tumors. The most common type is the granulosa-cell tumor. Because this type of tumor produces hormones, women tend to become symptomatic when the disease is present at an early stage. These tumors can affect both ovaries in 4–26% of cases, which makes a complete surgical evaluation very important.

The overall prognosis for women with sex cord–stromal tumors is very good, particularly because women tend to report to doctors early with these tumors. However, even in cases of early disease, the tumor can come back. It's not uncommon for women to have their cancer return 5 to 20 years after their initial diagnosis, which is why close monitoring of women with such tumors is very important. These tumor cell types are included in **Table 3**.

Table 3   Sex cord–stromal tumors

Granulosa-cell tumor
Thecoma-fibroma
Fibroma
Sertoli-Leydig cell
Leydig cell
Sarcomatoid (undifferentiated)
Gynandroblastoma
Unclassified

9. Are there risk factors for ovarian cancer?

As with most other cancers, ovarian cancer likely arises from many factors and most likely is due to genetic damage that builds up over time. It is important to distinguish the difference between "genetic damage" and "hereditary damage" in this context. Changes to one's genes, called **mutations**, occur spontaneously as a simple, random mistake in cell growth, sometimes related to an environmental factor. Most mutations are harmless; many that are harmful nevertheless do no damage because they are eliminated by the body's immune system, but some are able to escape the immune system, replicate themselves, and form cancers. A small number of these cancer-causing mutations can be passed from parent to child. Approximately 10% of ovarian cancers are truly related to heredity; the vast majority (90%) of ovarian cancers happen because of random mutations, otherwise known as **sporadic** mutations.

Ovarian cancer likely arises from many factors and most likely is due to genetic damage that builds up over time.

Mutations

Genetic changes in DNA; mutations are not always harmful but sometimes can be associated with cancer development.

Sporadic

Isolated; to occur without a pattern.

Several factors are associated with an increased risk for ovarian cancer. The most common type of ovarian cancer—epithelial ovarian cancer—appears to be related to how many times a woman ovulates. Every time an egg is released, the ovarian surface has to be repaired; each time this happens, it creates a risk that genetic mutations will accumulate. This condition may lead to epithelial ovarian cancer. This hypothesis is supported by the fact that decreasing ovulation with the use of oral contraceptives is associated with a decreased risk of getting ovarian cancer in the future.

Other risk factors for ovarian cancer include older age, a family history of breast and ovarian cancer, and French-Canadian or Jewish/Eastern European decent. The use of hormone replacement therapy (HRT) is not considered a risk factor (see Question 10). The use of fertility drugs for women having trouble becoming pregnant has been debated as a possible risk for increased ovarian cancer, but no evidence concludes that these medications cause ovarian cancer.

10. Is hormone replacement therapy associated with ovarian cancer?

Hormone replacement therapy (HRT) has been used in women for several decades as a way to control the symptoms of menopause. The main reason for using HRT currently is to help women deal with hot flashes and night sweats associated with menopause. Although long-term use of HRT has been associated with a slightly increased risk of breast cancer, HRT's association with ovarian cancer is less clear.

The main symptoms of ovarian cancer are bloating, abdominal pain, and distension.

11. What are the symptoms of ovarian cancer?

The main symptoms of ovarian cancer are bloating, abdominal pain, and distension. A recent study from the University of California at Irvine compared the prior symptoms and testing of women who were eventually diagnosed with ovarian cancer with those of women who did not have a cancer diagnosis and to a third group of women diagnosed with breast cancer. The researchers showed that the specific symptoms of bloating and abdominal pain were more likely in women diagnosed with ovarian cancer and represented "target symptoms." More importantly, they showed that these symptoms were present as many as 6 months prior to the diagnosis of ovarian cancer. On the basis of this work and prior research like it, we feel a woman should be cautioned that if she develops bloating, an increase in her waistline not due to a change in eating habits, lower abdominal discomfort, or pelvic pain, she should seek consultation with a physician. A work-up should include pelvic imaging and a CA-125, especially if the symptoms are unexplained.

Occasionally, women have shortness of breath that can be misinterpreted as a heart or lung problem; actually, it may be due to a buildup of fluid in the lung (a **pleural effusion**). Acid reflux, constipation, nausea, or vomiting may also be obvious, particularly when associated with early sensations of fullness at meals or a generally decreased appetite.

Pleural effusion
Fluid build-up around the lungs.

Women with germ-cell tumors often go to their doctor with abdominal pain that persists over several days or weeks and are also found to have a palpable (touchable) pelvic mass when examined. If the mass twists on itself or undergoes **torsion**, it can cause immediate and often unbearable pain. Such a mass can also cause pain due to bleeding or if it ruptures. These cancers typically grow very rapidly and at surgery can be as large as 40 centimeters. Fortunately, 70% of women with germ-cell tumors will be diagnosed with early-stage disease.

Torsion
Act of twisting or turning in on itself (ovarian torsion, for example).

Sex cord–stromal tumors appear early owing to their production of hormones, and their appearance can range from early puberty in young girls to postmenopausal bleeding in mature women. Abnormal vaginal bleeding is a common reason for women with granulosa-cell tumors to see their doctor. Other ways the disease can show up is by a mass felt on physical examination, ovarian torsion, rupture, or hemorrhage. Thecomas (tumors of theca cells) actively secrete hormones, and women seek a doctor owing to the effects of too much estrogen. Women with Sertoli-cell tumors also go to their doctor for the same reason, although they may have high blood pressure from excess production of a kidney hormone—called **renin** —necessary for blood pressure regulation. Fifty percent of women with Sertoli-Leydig-cell tumors notice symptoms related to too many androgens, or male hormones, which can cause a decrease in breast tissue or male-pattern baldness.

12. What is ascites? What causes it? How do you treat it?

Ascites is the build-up of fluid in the **peritoneal cavity**. The peritoneum is a sac made of a thin layer of tissue that lines the abdominal cavity and covers most of our internal abdominal and pelvic organs and the intestines. Ascites is a hallmark of advanced ovarian carcinoma and it is very commonly seen in patients with disease that has spread outside of the ovary to involve the peritoneum or other organs in the abdomen. Ascites can develop for numerous reasons; however, in the setting of ovarian cancer the most likely explanation is the spread of disease to organs inside the abdomen, the omentum, and the diaphragm. Ascites may be formed due to noncancerous conditions such as liver disease or heart failure, but in the setting of ovarian cancer, ascites is most commonly considered "malignant ascites." Ascites may accumulate to a large volume; some patients may have several liters of this usually amber-colored fluid inside the abdomen, which causes distention and may be the presenting symptom of ovarian carcinoma. Women with ascites may complain of discomfort, indigestion, and sometimes difficulty breathing due to pressure on the diaphragm.

Treatment of ascites usually consists of a combination of a drainage procedure followed by chemotherapy. A drainage of the ascites can be performed by **paracentesis**, a bedside procedure done under a local anesthetic to the abdominal wall. A small needle is introduced through the skin into the peritoneal cavity and connected to a vacuum bottle, where

Renin

A hormone released by the kidney normally that is important in maintaining hydration.

Ascites

Fluid build-up within the abdomen.

Peritoneal cavity

The abdominal space.

Paracentesis

The process of removing ascites.

the fluid is drained from the abdomen. Several liters of fluid can be removed this way with almost immediate symptom relief. Ascites also can be drained at the time of a surgical procedure for the cancer. However, if the patient does not receive chemotherapy promptly, ascites is very likely to reaccumulate within several days. The majority of patients with new ovarian cancer (70–80%) will respond to chemotherapy, and chemotherapy will usually prevent reaccumulation of ascites. Chemotherapy can be given either intravenously or sometimes through a semi-permanent catheter placed into the peritoneal cavity where chemotherapy washes are given directly into the peritoneum.

If the cancer does not respond to initial chemotherapy or returns after some time and starts to grow once more, your belly may fill up with ascites again. In that event, doctors use other types of chemotherapy to get control of your cancer, which is the primary way to control the ascites. If the swelling continues to recur, your physician may repeat the paracentesis multiple times.

13. What about pleural effusions? How do you treat them?

A pleural effusion is the build-up of fluid within the lung cavity, which is lined by a thin membrane of tissue called the pleura that envelops the lungs and the inner lining of the chest wall. Pleural effusions are occasionally seen with cases of advanced ovarian carcinoma. Like ascites, pleural effusions may be related to other medical conditions such as inflammation, infection, or heart disease. In the setting of advanced ovarian cancer, it may be an extension of advanced ascites related to advanced stage cancer. A large pleural effusion may cause shortness of breath and sometimes causes difficulty breathing (**dyspnea**).

Dyspnea
Shortness of breath.

The treatment of a pleural effusion will depend on the size of the effusion and the patient's symtoms. A moderate or large symptomatic pleural effusion that is causing symptoms of

19

Thoracentesis

Procedure of draining a pleural effusion.

shortness of breath will usually require drainage. This procedure, called a **thoracentesis**, can be performed as a bedside procedure. A needle is introduced under local anesthesia between the ribs to aspirate the fluid from the chest and allow the lung tissue to expand and provide more room for breathing. This will usually result in immediate and significant improvement in breathing and less discomfort to the patient.

Thoracic surgeon

A surgeon who has completed extra training in the surgical management of diseases involving the chest and its organs.

Pleurodesis

Process performed to prevent further build-up of fluid around the lung.

Alternatively, a pleural effusion can also be treated by placement of a chest tube. A small incision is made between the ribs and a small tube is introduced into the chest cavity and connected to a special suction device; this drains the fluid from the pleural cavity continuously and allows re-expansion of the lung over several days. The advantage of chest tube placement is that it allows the drainage of a large amount of effusion over several days. It also allows the **thoracic surgeon** to introduce a chemical substance into the lung for a procedure called **pleurodesis,** where a chemical substance such as talc is used to seal the pleura and hopefully prevent reaccumulation of malignant pleural effusion in the future.

Similar to malignant ascites in the peritoneal cavity, the ultimate treatment for a malignant pleural effusion will be effective systemic chemotherapy that will reduce the bulk of the tumor or completely eliminate the tumor. This will provide the patient with the best likelihood of the fluid not reaccumulating in the future.

14. What tests are used to diagnose ovarian cancer? How is a cancer diagnosis determined from these tests?

Ovarian cancer is diagnosed at surgery. Prior to surgery, tests that may help to make the diagnosis include a pelvic ultrasound (to check the size and nature of the ovaries) and a CT scan of the abdomen and pelvis. Such a scan can show a pelvic mass and also describe the presence of ascites (fluid buildup) and the possibility of **peritoneal carcinomatosis** or liver involvement. An MRI (magnetic resonance imaging) of the pelvis is also helpful to describe the nature of any pelvic abnormality, especially how deeply involved a tumor is with its surroundings.

The main diagnostic tool for ovarian cancer, however, remains surgery. All the imaging tests described previously can suggest ovarian cancer. However, the tumor has to be removed, seen under a microscope, and examined by a pathologist to confirm the diagnosis.

To make a diagnosis of cancer, a pathologist looks for specific features in a cell. Some of the criteria that influence a decision are (1) changes in the cell that make it appear different from a normal appearance, otherwise known as **atypia**; (2) intact or distorted architecture of the cell; and (3) evidence that the cell is dividing actively, also known as **mitosis**. A pathologist can also look for evidence of spread, or **metastases**, through the microscope by examining other tissue, such as the lymph nodes.

A pathologist looking at an ovarian tumor may see the cancer cells starting to pass through blood channels (**capillaries**) or lymph channels within the tissue; that may signal an increased risk for metastasis. In some instances, the pathologist can make a diagnosis of cancer without needing to look at the tumor. If fluid was surrounding the lung (pleural effusion) or was present within the abdomen (ascites), analyzing the fluid for cancer cells (known as cytology) could be sufficient to make a diagnosis of cancer.

15. What is the CA-125 test and what is its purpose?

The CA-125 is a blood test that can be used in the management of ovarian cancer. It measures a protein (called an **antigen**) that

Peritoneal carcinomatosis
Involvement of the omentum or bowels with cancer, usually the size of "rice granules" or tumor nodules.

Atypia
Used by pathologists, it describes abnormal cellular changes seen under the microscope.

Mitosis
Process of cells dividing.

Metastases
Tumor that has spread to distant places in the body.

Capillaries
The smallest blood vessels within your body.

Antigen
A protein that sits on or is released from cells that can be targeted with an antibody or a vaccine.

is found in your bloodstream. It is a carbohydrate molecule (hence the CA, which stands for **carbohydrate antigen**).

Carbohydrate antigen

A type of protein released from cells.

This test has been available for many years but isn't considered a useful test to diagnose ovarian cancer. "Normal" CA-125 varies from woman to woman, so the measurement isn't an absolute, and fluctuations in the CA-125 level are common: It might be elevated during one doctor's visit but be below normal 4 weeks later. Such changes in the CA-125 suggest that other factors not related to ovarian cancer—such as endometriosis, pelvic inflammatory disease, and uterine fibroids, to name a few—can influence the CA-125 level. The CA-125 level is useful to help follow women who are being treated or have been treated for ovarian cancer and whose CA-125 was high at the time of diagnosis. That is, the levels of this antigen compared to previous measurements can be used as an indicator of what might be happening with the patient's ovarian cancer. If the CA-125 results remain low and within normal limits, it's usually a good sign that the disease is not back or growing. However, if the CA-125 value starts to rise beyond what the laboratory considers a normal value (in most labs, <35 mg/dL), a recurrence must be ruled out. Nevertheless, the CA-125 is not, and should not be, the only measurement for such tracking (or follow-up) in ovarian cancer.

The CA-125 may also be used in the initial evaluation of an ovarian cyst. A normal CA-125 result is often reassuring and may help your doctor decide to observe—as opposed to operate on—an ovarian cyst. However, if the CA-125 result is elevated, it may be evidence that your doctor uses to recommend that an ovarian cyst be surgically evaluated.

Remember that the CA-125 (as mentioned) is not a test specific only to ovarian cancer, and its results can be elevated in a variety of noncancerous conditions, such as endometriosis, uterine fibroids, inflammatory diseases, other cancers such as breast or lung cancer, and even menstruation. This limits the use of CA-125 in ovarian cancer screening.

16. Should I have a PET scan?

A PET (positron emission tomography) scan is a test that allows doctors to evaluate metabolic processes, and most commonly tracks sugar (glucose) metabolism. When cells become cancerous, there can be a detectable increase in their use of glucose, making PET a potentially valuable tool in the evaluation, staging, and tracking of cancer. It is used in the management of multiple tumors including breast, lung, and colorectal cancers. Its role in ovarian cancer continues to be explored and we do not routinely use it in women with ovarian cancer. Small studies suggest that PET scans can predict response as early as 2 weeks into treatment with chemotherapy, but these results have yet to be tested in larger groups of women. Given the lack of evidence that PET scans can help improve outcomes in women with ovarian cancer, we feel it is investigational and not ready for use outside of clinical trials.

17. What is staging? How is ovarian cancer staged?

When you have surgery to remove an ovarian tumor, the surgeon will also check to see whether the cancer has spread throughout the abdomen and pelvis. This process is known as surgical staging (see **Table 4**).

Surgery for ovarian cancer requires a **laparotomy,** a vertical incision in the abdomen starting from the pubic area and extending to the belly button. The surgery requires removal of the omentum, the fatty tissue that drapes between the stomach and colon; removal of lymph nodes from the pelvis and around the largest artery in the body, known as the aorta; and obtaining multiple tissue specimens (**biopsies**) from the right and left sides of the pelvis, from the right and left sides of the abdomen, and from both diaphragms. In addition, surgeons would obtain washings from the abdomen to assess for floating cancer cells. The appendix might also be removed. The pelvic part of the procedure requires removal of both tubes

Laparotomy

Surgery through a large incision in the abdomen.

Biopsy

Removal of a small amount of tissue for analysis by a pathologist. It can be done during surgery or before surgery using other less invasive procedures.

Table 4   FIGO staging system of ovarian cancer

Stage	Definition
I	Cancer is limited to one or both ovaries.
IA	Cancer is limited to one ovary, and the tumor is confined to the inside of the ovary, without evidence of cancer on the outer surface. No ascites is present, and the ovarian surface is intact.
IB	Cancer is limited to both ovaries without any tumor on their outer surfaces. No ascites is present, and the surface of the tumor is unruptured.
IC	Tumor meets the criteria for either stage IA or stage IB, but one or more of the following are present: (1) tumor is present on the outer surface of one or both ovaries; (2) at least one of the ovarian surfaces has been seen to rupture (or ruptures during the process of removing it); or (3) ascites or abdominal washings are noted and contain malignant cells.
II	The tumor involves one or both ovaries with extension to other pelvic structures.
IIA	The cancer has extended to and/or involves the uterus or the fallopian tubes or both.
IIB	The cancer has extended to the bladder or rectum.
IIC	The tumor meets criteria for either stage IIA or stage IIB, and ascites or abdominal (peritoneal) washings contain malignant cells.
III	The tumor involves one or both ovaries, and one or both of the following are present: (1) The cancer has spread beyond the pelvis to the lining of the abdomen, or (2) the cancer has spread to the lymph nodes. The tumor is limited to the true pelvis but with histologically proven malignant extension to the small bowel or omentum.
IIIA	No cancer is grossly visible in the abdomen, and it has not spread to the lymph nodes. However, when biopsies are checked through a microscope, very small deposits of cancer are found in the abdominal (peritoneal) surfaces, also known as microscopic metastases.
IIIB	Deposits of cancer large enough for the surgeon to see but not exceeding 2 cm in diameter are present in the abdomen. The cancer has not spread to the lymph nodes.
IIIC	The cancer has spread to lymph nodes and/or the deposits of cancer exceed 2 cm in diameter and are found in the abdomen.
IV	Growth of the cancer involves one or both ovaries, and distant metastasis to the liver or lungs has occurred. Finding ovarian cancer cells in the excess fluid accumulated around the lungs (pleural fluid) is also evidence of stage IV disease.

FIGO = Federation International de Gynecologie et d'Obstetrique (International Federation of Gynecologic Oncologists).

and ovaries and the uterus (**bilateral salpingo-oophorectomy** and **total hysterectomy**).

Very few women get ovarian cancer before menopause, so retaining fertility is not a concern for nearly 90% of ovarian cancer patients—but there are occasionally younger women, like Andrea, who are diagnosed with cancer before menopause. In selected patients who strongly want to have children some day and in whom no visible disease is seen outside the ovaries at the time of surgery, a fertility-sparing operation could be performed (see Question 26).

The staging system is based on the findings at the time of surgery. Table 4 gives the staging system created by the International Federation of Gynecologic Oncologists (FIGO).

18. What is the "grade" of a cancer? Is it the same thing as the "stage"?

The **grade** is not the same thing as the stage of a cancer. Staging is a way of describing the location and spread of cancer. The staging system for ovarian cancer requires surgery to determine the extent of disease. The grade of cancer, on the other hand, is a way of describing the cells themselves in comparison to normal cells—a means of saying just how abnormal an abnormal cell appears.

Table 4 describes the staging system in detail. In general, stage I disease is limited to the ovary; stage II cancer will have spread from the ovary to other pelvic organs; stage III cancer has spread to abdominal surfaces, lymph nodes, and intestinal surfaces; and stage IV cancer will have spread to the liver, the lungs, or other distant places. The staging system serves several purposes. First, it provides a standard language so that all of the people involved in treatment of ovarian cancer, from the surgeon to the medical oncologist to the nurses, can understand the extent of disease when a woman presents with ovarian cancer. Second, it is used to decide what kind of treatment is used. Finally, it's used when we try to determine

Bilateral salpingo-oophorectomy
The surgical term for removal of both the right and left fallopian tubes and ovaries.

Total hysterectomy
Surgical excision of the uterus and cervix.

Grade
A pathologist term that defines how abnormal a cell is under the microscope.

Well-differentiated

A pathologist's term to describe cellular changes of a cancer cell; this describes cells that meet the criteria for cancer but still maintain a resemblance to normal cells.

Moderately differentiated

A pathologist's term to describe cellular changes of a cancer cell; cells that do not resemble their normal appearance but are still recognizable as related to their normal counterparts.

Poorly differentiated

A pathologist's term to describe cellular changes of a cancer cell; this describes cells that bear no resemblance to their normal counterparts.

In some cancers, including ovarian cancer, the grade can be used to predict how well your cancer will respond to chemotherapy.

the chances that you may have in beating the cancer (your prognosis).

The grade of a cancer, on the other hand, tells us something quite different. As mentioned in Question 14, the degree of cellular change, or atypia, is an important factor in determining normal from abnormal cells. Pathologists use a scoring system to determine how greatly these cells differ from their normal counterparts; that's termed the grade. In this system, grade I cancers are very similar to normal tissue and are called **well-differentiated**. As cancers look increasingly abnormal, their grade gets higher. Thus, grade II cancers are **moderately differentiated**; grade III cancers are **poorly differentiated**; and grade IV cancers, which bear no resemblance to normal tissue, are undifferentiated.

In some cancers, including ovarian cancer, the grade can be used to predict how well your cancer will respond to chemotherapy. Grade I tumors are slow-growing and are not as responsive to chemotherapy, but grade III tumors usually respond well because they are much more active and dividing.

19. What is my prognosis, and how is it determined?

A prognosis is an assessment of how a person diagnosed with a specific disease is likely to do and gives an estimate of the likelihood of cure or long-term survival. It is based on the information we have learned over the years about how women with the various stages and grades of ovarian cancer do over time. It is not something that is carved in stone; cancer patients with poor prognoses (i.e., the dreaded statement, "You have six months to live") have been known to do far better than predicted, with some surviving years, even decades, longer than forecast by their prognoses. Every patient is different, and your response to a particular form of treatment may be better or worse than average, so take the prognosis with a grain of salt.

The prognosis of patients with ovarian cancer depends on a variety of factors. Some important factors that have an impact on prognosis are (1) the type of cancer as determined through the microscope, (2) the stage of ovarian cancer, (3) whether all visible cancer was removed at surgery, (4) the size of any disease left after the initial surgery, and (5) your overall medical condition and age.

The prognosis is generally good for stage I ovarian cancer. One recent study indicated that women with stage I ovarian cancer who had a preoperative CA-125 below 30 U/mL and underwent complete surgical evaluation for their disease had a very good prognosis, and may not need further treatment beyond surgery. However, it is still not clear which individual or group of patients can be spared chemotherapy, and a fraction of patients will still require additional treatment in the form of chemotherapy after surgery.

For more advanced stages, the prognosis will depend on the results of the initial surgery. The best surgical result is to leave no visible disease at the end (otherwise known as a **complete resection**). Patients with no visible remaining (residual) disease tend to have a prognosis and overall survival rate better than those of patients whose disease cannot be completely removed. If visible residual disease cannot be completely removed, it is best to leave behind the smallest amount of disease. Patients who have disease less than 1 centimeter in diameter at the end of surgery (otherwise known as **optimal debulking**) do better than those who have disease greater than 1 centimeter (also called a **suboptimal debulking**).

Sometimes in advanced ovarian cancer, a tumor larger than 1 centimeter may be located in close proximity to vital structures, such that attempts to completely remove it would cause significant injury and/or lead to permanent disfigurement or disability. In such cases, surgeons would still require chemotherapy to fight the disease left behind.

Complete resection

Removal of all the tumor in your abdomen and pelvis.

Optimal debulking

Surgical result if residual tumor is less than 1 cm in diameter at the end of surgery.

Suboptimal debulking

Residual disease greater than 1 cm in diameter upon completion of surgery.

20. How does ovarian cancer spread? Does it usually spread to particular locations?

The most dangerous type of ovarian cancer—or any cancer—is cancer that has metastasized, or spread to another part of the body. The danger lies in the fact that once cancer metastasizes, it can go just about anywhere and start growing new tumors. Like other cancers, ovarian cancer that metastasizes can show up in the lungs, liver, or even the brain. However, for reasons not fully understood, this cancer seems to "prefer" the environment of the abdomen and pelvis and will most often grow and spread in these areas, even when it recurs.

Like other cancers, ovarian cancer that metastasizes can show up in the lungs, liver, or even the brain.

Ovarian cancer can spread (metastasize) in one of three ways. In local extension, the cancer can spread locally, either by growing directly on the surface of adjacent tissue (**direct extension**) or by growing through the surface of the peritoneum, the inner lining of your abdomen. When it spreads by such direct extension, the cancer attaches and then spreads to the fallopian tube, uterus, bladder, peritoneum, or rectal surface. This is a common way for locally advanced disease to spread. The other way is by spreading along the peritoneum. Ovarian cancer can shed from its original site in the ovary and land anywhere on the lining of the pelvic or abdominal peritoneum, where it can form new tumor nodules covering the lining of the pelvis or the lining of the abdomen or even replacing the omentum (the normal fatty structure that drapes between the stomach and transverse colon). This is a very common site in which to find advanced ovarian cancer. When the omentum is replaced with tumor, it is commonly described as an **omental cake**.

Direct extension

The process by which cancer extends into local and surrounding tissue.

Omental cake

Tumor involvement of the omentum that results in the formation of a large mass.

Lymphatic channels

Vessels through which lymph fluid travels; part of the lymphatic system.

Another path for metastasis lies through the **lymphatic channels**. Lymphatic channels form a complex and extensive network of channels found throughout the body. They function to drain the body of waste. Ovarian carcinoma can spread through the lymph nodes of the pelvis into the periaortic area and occasionally can even spread to lymph nodes in the chest and neck region. Approximately 20% of apparent early ovarian cancer may have disease spread outside the ovary, particularly in lymph nodes. With advanced ovarian cancer, the lymph nodes may be involved in as many as 60% of patients.

Metastasis can also take place through the bloodstream. When cancer invades into blood vessels, it can travel throughout the body, a process called **hematogenous dissemination**. It is through the bloodstream that ovarian cancer spreads to the lungs, liver, or brain.

Hematogenous dissemination

A process of spreading by which cancer travels through the bloodstream.

21. What sort of doctor should I consult? Should I get a second opinion? Could consulting another doctor affect my treatment or prognosis?

Choosing your doctor is ultimately a decision that can affect your outcome and your survival. Your primary physician probably handled matters through your initial diagnosis, and indeed may be a good person to assist you throughout your treatment. However, even if he or she is a gynecologist, your primary physician probably is not a specialist in treating ovarian cancer and therefore cannot be expected to be up to date on the latest information about this disease. Moreover, you are going to need surgery to remove the cancer, and that's something your primary physician cannot provide—but a **gynecologic oncologist** can. Thus, your outcome and chances of survival may be improved if you request from the beginning that a gynecologic oncologist be involved in your care, either as your primary surgeon or as a standby assistant surgeon. If you're diagnosed with ovarian cancer by your primary physician, please seek consultation with a gynecologic oncologist as soon as possible.

Choosing your doctor is ultimately a decision that can affect your outcome and your survival.

Gynecological oncologist

A specialist in the treatment of cancer of the female reproductive system.

You could also request a referral to a gynecologic oncologist to obtain a second opinion if you wish to be absolutely certain about the nature of your illness or the type of cancer and its treatment options. A second opinion is always reasonable. In general, a second opinion is a good idea if surgery has been recommended, because the type and extent of the surgical procedure can affect overall treatment recommendations and may even alter your prognosis. Women who have all their cancer removed (complete resection) or have all but less than 1 centimeter of disease removed (optimal debulking) tend to fare better than do women whose cancer cannot be removed for technical reasons (suboptimal debulking). In general, a qualified gynecological oncologist, not a general surgeon or gynecologist, should perform any surgery for ovarian cancer.

A second opinion is a good idea if surgery has been recommended.

When it comes to chemotherapy, a second opinion is reasonable if you are interested in a clinical trial (discussed in Question 41) or a more aggressive approach beyond what is done routinely. Ongoing research is trying to improve on the results of standard treatment, and you should explore such research if you are interested. If a cancer comes back (recurs), a second opinion is very reasonable in order to explore clinical trials and the different ways to treat recurrent disease.

PART THREE

Treatment of Ovarian Cancer

How do I decide on where to be treated?

Who's involved in my treatment?

Who should do my surgery?

More...

22. How do I decide where to be treated?

Deciding where to obtain treatment is a very personal issue, and your comfort with your treating physician should guide you. Your relationship with your oncologist is going to be one of the most important relationships you have; for that reason, it must be based on trust and honesty. If you do not feel comfortable asking questions or you feel that your oncologist is not taking you seriously, you should find a new provider. Just as important is that your oncologist be accessible. Chemotherapy causes side effects that can require frequent visits to your doctor's office or may require you to go into a hospital. The distance you have to travel should also be a factor to consider. The worst situation is to feel sick but helpless because you live too far away.

23. Who's involved in my treatment?

It's important for you to be treated with a team of specialists that should include a medical oncologist, a surgical oncologist (preferably one who specializes in gynecologic oncology; see Question 21), a radiation oncologist, and a pathologist. The pathologist is important because this person will confirm your cancer diagnosis and help to stage (define the extent of) the disease.

For women with ovarian cancer, the gynecological oncologist may take on a double role as both surgical and medical oncologist. For others, the surgeon and the medical oncologist will work closely together. The radiation oncologist is a specialist in the use of radiation to treat cancer; although it has a limited role in women newly diagnosed, radiation may become important for women with recurrent cancer.

In addition to these physician specialists, it is important to have access to the supporting staff in the office, including but not limited to the oncology nurses, social workers, and clinical therapists who can help you and your loved ones adjust to often difficult situations.

Assembling a medical team and support network is crucially important. Healing takes place on many levels, known and unknown, and I think that one step toward health is choosing and having confidence in your medical team. Another is realizing and accepting the responsibility that you have as part of that team. Ultimately, the patient is the one to make the decisions and, in my case, I rely on the doctors to present options to work with. Fighting cancer is a Herculean task, and you want your support staff to be the best you can find. Don't give up until you find people with whom you can work, from whom you can learn, and in whom you can have confidence.

Sometimes it's helpful to enlist the opinion of family and friends, and some of the most positive feedback I heard was from someone who initially told me to know that I deserved to get the best care and not to be afraid to ask for it. Being sick at times made me feel very vulnerable and dependent, and I am thankful that I was always reminded that I was an integral part of the medical team: It made me feel more confident and in control of a situation that was unknowable and chaotic. And I learned a lot when a friend prayed with me before a major surgery, asking God to guide the surgeon's hands. —Andrea Brown

SURGERY

24. Who should do my surgery?

If a diagnosis of ovarian cancer is suspected or if the possibility of ovarian cancer is present, surgery is best performed by a gynecologic oncologist. Gynecologic oncologists are physicians who have completed a full training in general obstetrics and gynecology and have received additional specialized training in gynecologic oncology (usually 2–4 years).

Surgery for ovarian cancer is best performed where the appropriate operation can be conducted and resection of advanced disease can be as complete as possible. Unfortunately, many patients with ovarian cancer continue to have their surgery performed by non-oncologic surgeons; this results in an incomplete operation or a less aggressive attempt at resection. In such situations, a patient may require additional surgery in order to stage the disease completely or to resect advanced disease.

25. What will the surgeon do?

The first things that the surgeon will do are study your medical history; perform a thorough examination, including a pelvic examination; and review any radiology studies. If the history review and examination suggest ovarian cancer, your surgeon will recommend surgery. The goals of surgery are to remove the primary cancer, to determine whether the cancer has spread, and to attempt to remove the spread of cancer as best as possible.

Surgery for Apparently Early Disease

If radiology exams indicate that you have localized or early ovarian cancer (generally meaning the disease is contained only within your pelvis), the surgeon will remove both your tubes and ovaries and your uterus. That's described as a total abdominal hysterectomy and bilateral salpingo-oophorectomy. In addition, your surgeon will take samples from any areas of possible tumor spread as part of the staging procedure. That would mean taking the lymph nodes from both sides of your pelvis and around the aorta, removal of the omentum, and obtaining tissue from around your abdomen and pelvis (known as peritoneal biopsies) and washings to exclude cancer spread. If disease is present in your abdomen at the time of surgery, the goal of surgery would be to debulk or resect as much as possible, leaving the smallest possible amount of visible disease.

Advanced Disease

When ovarian cancer is advanced or widespread, more extensive surgery is usually needed, and you would likely undergo radical debulking. It is important to know that the description that follows applies only to selected patients with advanced bulky disease; it is not what early-stage ovarian cancer patients

undergo. However, it provides ample reason for a newly diagnosed patient to avoid delaying treatment.

Debulking usually requires a resection of the uterus, both
tubes and ovaries, possibly the rectum, and part of the large
colon. If that were the case, you might require a segment of
bowel pulled through your abdomen so that stool can drain (a
colostomy). This intestinal diversion is usually temporary and
may be reversed by another operation at a later date.

Occasionally, segments of small intestine have to be removed.
The lining of the abdomen may have implants on it, and these
are also removed. Occasionally, the lining of the diaphragm
also will have to be removed.

Less frequently, patients may have advanced disease involving their liver or gallbladder; in such cases, resection of these
areas may become necessary. The spleen is another organ
that occasionally can be involved in ovarian cancer. It is not
uncommon for women to undergo a splenectomy in order to
remove disease that may be involving the spleen. Occasionally, the appendix is removed as part of ovarian cancer surgery.
The overall intent is to completely remove all visible sites of
disease, leaving the abdomen and pelvis with the smallest
amount of residual tumor.

If a surgeon finds the disease is too advanced and cannot
be completely removed, or a woman's overall health makes
surgery highly risky, then primary treatment may consist of
chemotherapy, sometimes called **neoadjuvant treatment**. It is
used sometimes when your surgeon thinks you have a large
tumor burden that can't be completely removed. This approach
aims to decrease the volume of cancer so as to improve the
chances of optimal debulking (resection, or removal). If this
is the case, there may be a role for interval surgical debulking,
usually performed after three cycles of chemotherapy. A large
clinical trial of women compared those who had an initial
attempt at debulking and then were randomized to chemotherapy versus those who had chemotherapy for three cycles

Colostomy

A loop of bowel that
is pulled through
your skin.

*The overall
intent is to
completely
remove all
visible sites of
disease.*

**Neoadjuvant
treatment**

Treatment given
before surgery.

followed by surgery and more chemotherapy afterwards; no survival advantage was seen with interval surgery. Still, it was not any less successful, either.

26. Must the surgeon remove both ovaries if I am diagnosed with ovarian cancer?

Most ovarian cancer patients are postmenopausal, so concerns about fertility are irrelevant in the majority of cases. Some patients, however, are diagnosed before menopause, and a certain proportion of them, like Andrea, are concerned about maintaining their ability to have children in the future. If you have completed your family and have no desire to remain fertile, the standard of care is to remove both your ovaries and tubes and your uterus and to perform a staging operation. This has been the traditional surgical method of treating ovarian cancer, and it is the most likely method to prevent future recurrence. However, if you strongly desire to preserve your ability to have children and have no obvious spread of cancer outside your ovary, it may possible to retain your uterus and the uninvolved tube but proceed with a full staging operation. In that procedure, the uterus and the uninvolved tube and ovary are left intact and are not removed, which would allow a woman to have children in the future. Yet even in the case of fertility-sparing surgery, the operation should still include a complete staging, which would include removal of the lymph nodes and the omentum and obtaining the peritoneal biopsies. It is not clear what risks a woman takes when she undergoes conservative surgery to preserve her chances of having or carrying a baby later. Results presented from the Memorial Sloan-Kettering Cancer show that selected women undergoing conservative surgery had similar long-term survival compared to women undergoing complete surgical treatment. However, the number of women studied was small and the subject requires further studies.

Maintaining fertility is not something most ovarian cancer patients must worry about, but it was a major concern for my husband and me. We had been married for only 1½ years when I was diagnosed. We had to weigh the benefits of waiting to have surgery until eggs could be extracted or to see whether it was possible to retain an ovary against immediate and extensive surgery. One surgeon I consulted with asked if I wanted to wait a month in order to extract eggs (which we didn't, as we felt time was of the essence and wanted surgery as soon as possible); one explained to us that, given his experience with the disease and the factor of my age (39), he could only really advise removing both ovaries. My husband encouraged me to see another doctor, who said that he could see a possibility of keeping an ovary and the uterus intact if I was in early stage. This was one factor informing my choice of surgeon. However, owing to the spread of the disease, I had a full hysterectomy.

It took me a long time to mourn the loss of fertility. This has been hard on us as a couple because we so greatly wanted children. We have talked about adoption but have decided for the time being to leave it be. Time has helped us to accept these changes and to look forward instead of looking back to what could have been. Psychotherapy, both individually and in couples counseling, has helped us. But it remains poignant to remember what was lost.
—Andrea Brown

27. How important is staging? What if I wasn't staged—should I go back to the operating room?

Surgical staging is extremely important if you are diagnosed with ovarian cancer. Staging is usually performed by an operation via an incision in the abdomen or sometimes by **laparoscopy**. Staging requires the evaluation of the pelvic and abdominal organs in the peritoneal cavity and retroperitoneum with multiple biopsies, washings, removal of lymph nodes, sampling of any suspicious areas in the abdomen, and removal of the omentum. Staging also requires that an evaluation of the chest with a chest x-ray or a CT scan be performed to ensure that the lungs are free of disease. If your

Laparoscopy

Camera-directed surgery done without creating a large incision in the abdomen.

cancer appears to be limited to the ovary (stage I disease), surgical staging gains more importance. Anywhere between 20% and 30% of women who appear to have disease limited to the ovary will be found to have microscopic or small volume disease outside the ovary when staged. This may profoundly affect their postsurgical treatment, particularly regarding chemotherapy options.

Today, in the United States, many centers will treat advanced stage III ovarian carcinoma that has been successfully removed (also known as an optimal cytoreduction) with a combination of intravenous and intraperitoneal chemotherapy. If an adequate staging is not performed, it will be unlikely that patients with stage III disease based on microscopic disease will be identified. If you have been diagnosed with ovarian cancer and were not staged at that time, the decision of whether you should go back for a second surgery will depend on what was found at that first operation. If the disease appeared to be extensive and the patient will need prompt initiation of systemic chemotherapy, it may not be absolutely necessary to return for restaging. Still, staging should be considered in all women diagnosed with ovarian cancer.

28. What is an intravenous MediPort? Should I get one?

Reservoir

A receptacle that holds fluid.

A MediPort is a device made up of a small elastic tube connected to a **reservoir** that can be placed in the body under local anesthesia. It allows us to give medications and chemotherapy intravenously. The reservoir is usually placed over the rib cage and below the right or left collar bone, or alternatively, it can be placed in the arm. These catheters or reservoirs can then be removed in the clinic when chemotherapy is completed, usually under local anesthesia, without much difficulty.

The catheters are introduced through a large vein deep in the chest and the reservoir is fixed to the chest wall under the skin. These MediPorts allow administration of intravenous fluids, medications, and chemotherapy and also allow for drawing of blood periodically. The advantage of the MediPort is that it will avoid multiple peripheral phlebotomy and venous sticks in the arms, and the central MediPort can be used for the majority of intravenous blood draws or administration of medication. These ports are usually placed by an interventional radiologist under local anesthesia or by a gynecologic oncologist or a surgeon in the operating room. The ports can be removed under local anesthesia, either bedside or in the outpatient office setting. If you have a difficult vein to access and you have a hard time having blood drawn or starting intravenous infusion, insertion of a venous MediPort may be a good option. This MediPort can be removed at the end of chemotherapy.

I had it done for my second round of treatment and am glad I did. I'd recommend it for any woman who either a) can only use one arm for treatment because of prior surgery, or b) has ever been told by a nurse or phlebotomist that she's "a hard stick." But I wish I'd had it put in my chest ("subclavian") rather than my upper arm because it restricted my arm use. It hurt when I lifted shopping bags, etc., and I wasn't able to do the (very moderate) weightlifting exercises I was used to (and had enough energy for).

Women being treated in the winter months might want to think about taking an old long-sleeved shirt to a tailor and having a snap or Velcro flap put in over the port site—the chemo equivalent of a nursing shirt. This will eliminate the need to wear short-sleeved or low-cut clothes, or change into a johnny, for treatment.
—Marsha Posusney

CHEMOTHERAPY

29. Does everyone with ovarian cancer need chemotherapy?

Chemotherapy is recommended for every patient with ovarian cancer except those with stage IA, grade 1 or grade 2 tumors. Grade 3 cancers, even at the earliest stages, are usually treated with chemotherapy. Recently reported data based on two large trials in women with early-stage disease suggested that the addition of chemotherapy to surgery improves overall survival by 8% and improves the chances of not having it come back by 11%, compared to surgery alone.

For all women with ovarian cancer who undergo chemotherapy, the current standard of care is to give six cycles of platinum-based therapy, regardless of stage. It is still not clear whether less treatment is as effective; hopefully, the results of ongoing clinical trials will help us answer this question. Recently, intriguing data were published suggesting that women with a normal CA-125 at diagnosis with early ovarian cancer do not require chemotherapy. This will need to be confirmed in a clinical trial, however, before we can rely on this information. For women with advanced disease, the standard recommendation is platinum-based chemotherapy.

30. What kind of chemotherapy is used to treat ovarian cancer?

Landmark clinical trials have established that standard treatment of newly diagnosed epithelial ovarian cancer uses a taxane-platinum combination. These drugs are described below. Other drugs used to treat recurrent ovarian cancer are addressed in Question 77 and listed in **Table 6**.

Platinum agents (carboplatin and cisplatin) are the drugs most active in treating ovarian cancer; they work by creating breaks in the DNA, leading eventually to cell death. They can be given either by vein or directly into the abdomen (**intraperitoneal** treatment). Although active against cancer cells, they also affect normally dividing cells, which accounts for some of their side effects (discussed later).

Taxanes (paclitaxel, docetaxel) work by blocking microtubules (tiny structures important in the process of cells dividing). Paclitaxel was the drug initially studied in clinical trials

Intraperitoneal
Into the abdomen.

involving ovarian cancer patients. It is given over 24 hours, if combined with cisplatin, or as a 3-hour infusion when given with carboplatin, which is the more common chemotherapy program used. Recently, a large European study confirmed that docetaxel is equivalent to paclitaxel, but has fewer long-term side effects than paclitaxel.

31. How is chemotherapy administered?

There are new and emerging options for the standard chemotherapy program for ovarian cancer. If your surgeon successfully removed all or most of your disease (optimal debulking) and you had Stage III ovarian cancer, an emerging standard is a combination of chemotherapy given into your vein (intravenously) and into your abdomen, known as intraperitoneal administration (a **belly wash**). A recently reported clinical trial showed that a combined treatment approach with both intravenous (IV) and intraperitoneal (IP) treatment can dramatically improve survival to over 5 years. The regimen is more complicated than intravenous treatment alone, however, and may require a hospital stay to get the treatment. You should consult with your doctor to see if he or she is comfortable with this way of giving chemotherapy. If not, it might be worthwhile to go to a specialized center where it is done.

Belly wash

Common term for an intraperitoneal treatment.

The IP route requires placement of a temporary catheter in your abdomen that's connected to a small plastic container (a reservoir) positioned underneath the skin, usually right on top of your lower rib cage. The reservoir can be accessed with a needle through the skin, which allows drugs to be given directly into your abdomen. The agents are allowed to spread throughout the peritoneal cavity (hence the term *belly wash*) and eventually are absorbed through the abdominal lining over the next 1 to 2 days. This method of administering chemotherapy is attractive for patients with ovarian cancer because this disease tends to spread through the lining of the abdomen and, in many cases, stays in the peritoneal cavity.

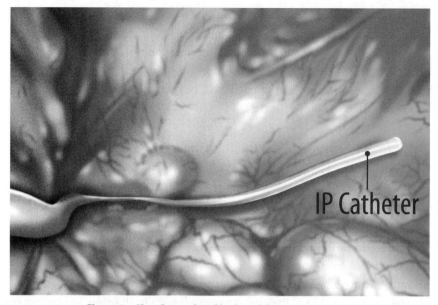

IP Catheter

Figure 4   IP catheter placed in the pelvis.

The IP catheter and reservoir are removed after the treatment is completed. This generally does not require a large surgery and is often performed in an outpatient setting under local anesthesia without much difficulty or complications. The IP catheter and reservoir, like any other foreign device in humans, carry a small risk of infection or malfunction, and occasionally the catheter has to be removed due to either malfunction or infection.

The main side effects during the treatment are feeling distended or cramping during administration of the chemotherapeutic agent. However, the drug can be absorbed into your bloodstream, and this can cause side effects.

Another standard option continues to be treatment by vein, which does not require you to stay in the hospital. This is still the standard of care for women whose cancers have spread beyond the abdomen (stage IV) or women with early disease (stage I or II).

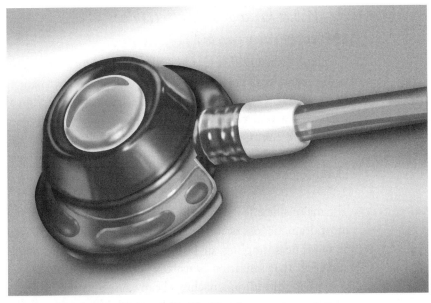

Figure 5   IP catheter and reservoir (BardPort type).

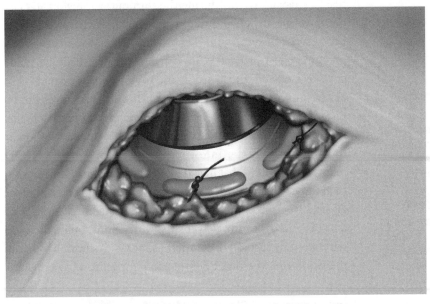

Figure 6   IP catheter reservoir placed under the skin over the left lower rib cage.

32. What kind of side effects does chemotherapy cause?

Cisplatin has significant side effects, including nausea and vomiting, potential hearing loss, kidney injury, and permanent nerve damage. Fortunately, we have learned through clinical trials that a very close cousin to cisplatin—carboplatin—is just as effective. Carboplatin is also less likely to injure the kidneys and nerves. Its major toxicity lies in decreasing your blood counts, which can make you prone to infection.

The major side effects of paclitaxel are total hair loss, with the most dramatic loss occurring after the first treatment, as well as numbness, tingling, or both, usually affecting the hands and feet. That sensation is usually reversible after paclitaxel is stopped. In addition, paclitaxel can cause a hypersensitivity reaction (your body reacting to what it thinks is a foreign substance) while the drug is being infused into your system. The reaction usually occurs during the start of the infusion and can occur during any of your treatments. It can be characterized by many types of symptoms: flushing, shortness of breath, chest pressure, chest or back pain, or rash. It can usually be managed by stopping the infusion and giving you an extra dose of **antihistamines**. Once the reaction subsides, paclitaxel can be restarted. This is because the reaction is caused not by paclitaxel itself but by the molecule with which it is mixed to allow it to be absorbed better into your bloodstream. Your body may react to this other substance (called a **cremaphore**) by releasing histamines that cause the reaction. Once your body releases all its histamines, the infusion can be restarted. In order to decrease the risk of hypersensitivity reactions, premedication with steroids (usually Dexamethasone) is used prior to treatment, starting the night before you get paclitaxel.

Docetaxel does not cause the same degree of numbness or tingling, although it does cause hair loss. Its major side effect is decreased blood counts, which can be treated with medications that boost blood cell production. Other side effects of

Antihistamine

To block the release of histamines, which are often associated with allergic reactions.

Cremaphore

A molecule to which drugs are attached to increase the drugs' delivery into your body.

docetaxel are hypersensitivity reactions and fluid build-up, which can cause your face, arms, or legs to swell. The risk for both of these side effects can be reduced with the use of steroid premedication.

Fatigue or tiredness is a common effect of treatment that can get worse as you approach the end of your treatment (i.e., the fifth and sixth treatments). This may last for a couple of months, but then you should slowly start to feel like yourself once it is completed.

Most other chemotherapy drugs have similar side effects, including effects on the bone marrow, causing anemia, low platelets, or lowering white cells (and making you at risk of infections). Some of the drugs commonly used to treat ovarian cancer, however, do have drug-specific side effects. Liposomal doxorubicin can cause a red, scaling, and sometimes painful rash that can affect the hands and feet, and is called a hand-foot syndrome. Gemcitabine can cause low-grade fevers the day after it is given or even difficulty breathing or pleural effusions. Etoposide and hexamethylamine are oral agents that cause nausea and vomiting as their major toxicity. Topotecan can cause nausea as well, but its major toxicity is on the bone marrow. **Table 6** in Question 77 outlines the drugs that are routinely used to treat ovarian cancer and summarizes the major side effects of treatment.

I think it's important to note that there are side effects from the chemo drugs but also side effects from the drugs used to counteract them. During my chemotherapy teaching, before I started treatment, I wasn't warned about the side effects of decadron, a steroid used as a premedication for paclitaxel. The steroids can delay the onset of symptoms from the chemotherapy drugs, so I had no loss of energy on the night of treatment or the next day. But when the steroids wore off, the chemo effects would hit: on day 3 I would wake up feeling really weak and lethargic. The nurses referred to this as the "breakthrough effect." What I thought was scary at first is that I would also "see spots" when my eyes were closed. I noticed

*it in the shower when shampooing my hair or washing my face.
But my vision was unaffected and this phenomenon would abate
after a few days.*

*I also developed some mild acne and a scalp condition which a der-
matologist I consulted thought was caused by the decadron. Lastly,
I think the decadron, along with the anti-nausea drug Zofran,
contributed to the stomach acid problems I had with carboplatin
and paclitaxel. I experienced mild stomach distress, but not nausea, and starting the day after treatment, I'd get a steady but dull
stomachache. Eating didn't particularly help it but if I didn't eat
(or chew on Tums when food wasn't available) every few hours the
pain would become spasmodic. I would get spasms if I consumed
something acidic, like tea, or something very spicy. I found that
even when taking prescription antacids, for the first week after
treatment I had to put food in my stomach every couple of hours
and couldn't drink even a low acid tea without some spasms. At
that time, on the nurses' advice, I was taking Zofran prophylactically two or three times a day for the first days after treatment, and
I also had constipation problems for which I took Colace.*

*With my second recurrence, I was treated with carboplatin and
gemcitabine. A nurse suggested that the Zofran could be causing
the constipation, so I stopped taking it, never got nauseous, and the
acid problems went away as well. It could be that the paclitaxel
itself causes acid problems that the gemcitabine doesn't (and I also
got much less decadron with the gemcitabine), but I'd recommend
that anyone with a history of stomach acid problems NOT take
Zofran prophylactically until they know they need it.*

*My most challenging side effect on carboplatin and paclitaxel was
bone/joint pain though, which started on day 3 and lasted through
day 5 for the first four cycles; in my last two, when I was getting
Neulasta, the pain took a couple of days longer to go away. Ben-
gay provided some relief, as did hot baths. But Tylenol didn't help
with these, and I can't take NSAIDs because of my stomach acid
problems, so at times I had to take Percocet. After the first cycle I
learned to just not make plans for these days.*

Lastly, insomnia. The chemo process itself is pretty anxiety-producing, not to mention the worries about survival. Sometimes I had trouble falling asleep, though more often it was waking up sometime between 2 and 4 a.m. and not being able to fall back asleep. My social worker recently suggested that this, too, is aggravated by decadron, but I'm not sure it was any better on the Carbo/Gemzar than the CarboTaxol. In any case, I tried several different things, but found that the best thing for waking during the middle of the night was Xanax; for difficulty getting to sleep some relaxation/visual imaging tapes usually helped and I only took a pill if they didn't.

Patients like me who are pill averse should know that they can cut most pills in half and not worry about becoming dependent on sleeping or anti-anxiety meds. I was able to wean myself from these pretty quickly after treatment ended."—Marsha Posusney

After having treatments for more than two years, there has been an array of differing effects. They vary with the different kind of chemotherapy drugs and each has had its own unique side effects. The most noticeable is hair loss—it can be devastating to wake up and find you are bald. Then there are the other side effects like nausea, constipation, and diarrhea. Most of these can be controlled by medications; it just takes some time to find the correct combination that will work for you. Being tired and weak are other side effects. Sleep sometimes helps but not always. Then there were the treatments where I felt fine, except for the skin problems like small blisters and peeling. Despite them, I would not have known I was having treatment had it not been for the inevitable IV drip of chemotherapy. The vein started to become less able for IV treatments, and after many of them, I elected to have a MediPort surgically implanted. There is always anxiety of unknown side effects when a new chemotherapy is introduced; however, I have always been advised of any side effects. There are times when I had leg cramps while relaxing, or the inability to get a good night's sleep. Then again, the symptoms were controlled by medicine. —Phyllis Hames

TREATMENT OF NONEPITHELIAL OVARIAN CANCER

33. When do germ-cell tumors require chemotherapy?

In women diagnosed with early-stage disease, postsurgical treatment using chemotherapy is usually reserved for those with any of the following types of tumors: embryonal carcinomas, endodermal sinus tumors, or mixed germ-cell tumors. Women with these types of tumors are at a high risk of relapse, so chemotherapy is given after surgery in the hope that the drugs will destroy any tumor cells that might remain after surgery and thus prevent recurrence. Chemotherapy is also given in women who have advanced germ-cell tumors or in whom tumors have returned.

The general treatment uses drugs different from those used for epithelial cancers. The most common regimen (program or schedule) is bleomycin, etoposide, and cisplatin (BEP). It has been shown to be very active in the treatment of germ-cell cancers. However, this regimen is not without risks, and the potential benefit of treatment has to be weighed against the side effects of the treatment. Because women with germ-cell tumors are typically young when they are diagnosed, these considerations should not be taken lightly.

The major side effects that need to be considered are damage from bleomycin to your lungs, which can happen during or after treatment and can lead to scarring (or pulmonary fibrosis); damage from cisplatin to your nerves and kidneys, which can be permanent; and a risk (although rare) from etoposide of causing leukemia later in life.

More than 90% of patients with germ-cell tumors will be cured after the BEP program. The number of treatments is generally three or four cycles given every 3 weeks, although your physician may recommend more if your disease has spread or if treatment has to be changed due to side effects that occur while you're on BEP.

34. Do all types of sex cord–stromal tumors require chemotherapy?

No, not all sex cord or stromal tumors require chemotherapy. Many of these tumors will require only surgery, but it's important that surgical staging be complete, particularly in women who want to keep their fertility.

Early-stage granulosa-cell tumors do not warrant treatment after surgery. Even for women with advanced disease, the benefit of postoperative treatment with radiation, chemotherapy, or hormones is not completely clear. In such a case, your oncologist may recommend no further treatment except regular visits to the office every 3 to 4 months.

Even when disease recurs, surgery is the preferred choice of treatment. Your oncologist may offer chemotherapy, but this decision is an individual choice based on how much cancer was found, the length of time before the cancer came back, and how strong you are at the time of the recurrence. If chemotherapy becomes necessary, the regimen of choice is BEP. The optimal management for women with recurrent or incompletely resected disease has not been established.

35. Is chemotherapy ever recommended for borderline tumors?

Chemotherapy has no standard role in treating borderline tumors. The major treatment is surgical. If the entire tumor is removed, particularly if it is found at an early stage, women with these tumors are generally cured. Even if the disease has spread outside your pelvis, all attempts at removing all visible disease afford the best chance of survival; chemotherapy may or may not be recommended. In general, chemotherapy is reserved for tumors that were incompletely removed surgically or else are found through the microscope to be invasive (which can signify a more aggressive tendency to the borderline tumor, or even actual cancer). If chemotherapy is warranted, the tumor is treated with carboplatin and paclitaxel, just as for ovarian cancer.

36. Are any tumor markers associated with these nonepithelial types of ovarian tumors?

CA-125 results are sometimes increased in women with borderline tumors.

For the germ-cell tumors, two types of proteins are often elevated. These are the human chorionic gonadotropin (or the hCG) and alpha-feto protein (AFP). The hCG is what is tested in a pregnancy test, but in this situation it is used to monitor the activity of both nongestational choriocarcinomas and dysgerminomas to treatment. AFP is a tumor marker as well, and is elevated in endodermal sinus tumors, immature teratoma, and the embryonal carcinomas.

The sex cord–stromal tumors can cause increased estrogen and progesterone levels but do not usually have a tumor marker. One exception is the granulosa-cell tumor, which secretes a protein known as inhibin. Other useful markers may include LDH and CA-125.

37. What happens if the CA-125 result isn't normal during chemotherapy?

The CA-125 reading should decrease gradually with treatment. Ideally, it should be normal after the third treatment, although this may depend on how high the CA-125 result was when you started treatment. If it is going down slowly, your doctor may recommend additional cycles of treatment, usually up to eight cycles. If the number flattens out or starts to rise, it may indicate that your cancer is not responding to the treatment. It is important that a repeat evaluation be performed in that situation, usually with a CT scan. Signs signaling that the disease isn't responding call for a change in plan, because more of the same treatment is unlikely to help you.

If your disease stops responding to up-front treatment, your doctor may describe your cancer as "primary platinum-refractory." In women with platinum-refractory disease, the cancer is not curable. Instead, the goal of further therapy becomes one of control. This approach is similar to that taken for women with recurrent ovarian cancer, particularly if the cancer comes back in a short time (within 3 months of stopping treatment). The management (handling) of recurrent and refractory cancers is discussed later in this book (see Part Six).

38. Does radiation play a role in treatment?

Although it's not considered a standard treatment for ovarian cancer, radiation is an effective means of treatment. It has fallen out of favor as **adjuvant** treatment (i.e., after surgery) because chemotherapy has been shown to be an effective means of therapy. When used after initial surgery, radiation is directed against the entire abdomen; this carries a risk of complications to your bowel and kidneys. Therefore, it's usually reserved for treatment of recurrent tumors, particularly in situations in which an isolated recurrence can be encompassed in one radiation field.

Adjuvant
Given after a primary procedure.

39. What does consolidation mean?

When used in the treatment of ovarian cancer, consolidation refers to additional treatment offered to women who, after completing surgery and chemotherapy, have no cancer detectable by examination, radiology studies, or CA-125. The goal of this extra treatment is to increase the odds that the cancer will not come back (recur). Another term that describes this extra treatment is *maintenance*.

At some medical centers, this extra treatment may consist of further chemotherapy administered by vein; at other select centers, an intraperitoneal approach is used, as described in Question 31.

A recently completed randomized trial has shown that extending paclitaxel treatment as a monthly treatment for a year results in a longer duration without the cancer progressing, compared to a regimen of paclitaxel given monthly for 3 months. The study was terminated early due to this positive result, but whether this translates into long-term survival remains unknown. Clinical trials continue to ask the question of the role of this extended treatment in women with ovarian cancer using more chemotherapy or immunologic approaches (such as vaccines).

OTHER THERAPIES

40. What is a vaccine?

When we were kids, we routinely received a series of shots to protect us from infections. Those were **vaccines**. However, the role of vaccines in the fight against ovarian cancer is an area of active research.

As they relate to cancer treatment, vaccines are a novel way of stopping cancer from spreading by teaching the body's immune system to recognize the tumor cells as foreign and kill them off. There are various preparations of vaccines: Some are based on an individual's specific tumor, others are based on common molecules found in a majority of ovarian cancers, and still others are directed against CA-125. All are in clinical development throughout the country and are being tested in a number of ways to learn how to use them in battling ovarian cancer. All vaccines are still considered investigational, and you generally can receive them only if you are participating in a clinical trial. One vaccine, MAb B43.13 (oregovomab, Ovarex), is currently in a phase III randomized trial across the country for women who have completed up-front treatment for stage III or IV ovarian cancer.

41. When should I consider a clinical trial?

Participating in clinical trials (studies using patients) is always an option for women in all phases of ovarian cancer, from initial diagnosis to relapse to second remission. However, the vast majority of women turn to clinical trials only after standard therapy has failed.

There are no guidelines in place as to when a patient should participate in a clinical trial. Before you begin investigating trial options, it is important to understand the different types of studies done in cancer research, because not all trials are the same, and you need to look for one that is suited to your circumstances.

The vast majority of women turn to clinical trials only after standard therapy has failed.

There are three basic types of clinical trials. Phase I trials are the earliest type of clinical trials. They are designed to test a new medication or treatment strategy, and often they are "first-in-human" studies involving only a small number of patients. The main purpose of these trials is to determine the best dose of a new drug or treatment to take into further development. This is done by starting at a low dose and gradually increasing it until side effects are seen. This leads us to the second goal of these early trials: to determine what kind of side effects are associated with the new treatment being tested. It's important to realize that although most phase I trials want to test whether the study drug can cause tumors to shrink, it is not the primary goal.

Once a phase I trial is completed, the next step in development of a new treatment is to define how active a drug is. That's the goal of a phase II trial. Unlike phase I trials, the majority of phase II trials are conducted to target specific diseases. In general, all patients enrolled in these studies are treated with the study medication.

If a drug or treatment looks promising in a phase II trial, the next step—a phase III trial—involves comparing it against an accepted treatment in a specific disease setting. The goal is to determine whether the treatment being tested is better than the current available treatment. These are usually run as randomized trials (participating patients are assigned randomly to a treatment). Neither they nor their doctors can select the treatment they'll receive. The results of these trials usually determine the standard of care for oncologists.

For women with newly diagnosed ovarian cancer, phase II and phase III trials are available nationally, either through research centers as single-institution studies (meaning that a certain type of treatment is being studied in only one place) or as part of a cooperative group trial (meaning that patients are being offered the trial in multiple places). For women with recurrent cancers of the ovary, both types of trials may be available. Many of the trials limit entry by the number of prior therapies, which are decided by the physicians and scientists studying the treatment.

Often, patients who have had two or three different treatments are excluded from the trial; although exclusion is a controversial subject (no one wants to be denied a treatment that could save her life), there are some legitimate concerns that cause investigators to refuse women previously treated with other medications access to the trial. For example, many chemotherapy regimens are toxic, not just to cancer cells, but to organs such as the liver or the kidneys. If the clinical trial drug is thought to be equally or more toxic, the investigators might be concerned that women with toxicity from prior therapy could get sicker, not healthier, by participating in the trial. Fortunately, these concerns are less significant in trials of the new targeted therapies, so women previously treated with other drugs can often be admitted into such trials. Nevertheless, this consideration is important because it may affect your options to receive standard treatments before you enter the study.

It's important to understand that the purpose of a clinical trial is to test a theory, in this case usually a question regarding the effectiveness of a new treatment strategy. If something is being tested in a clinical trial, its benefit is still unproven. It's never wrong to explore clinical trial options for any stage of ovarian cancer, however, and remember: All of the current standard therapies were once unproven—they only became standard therapies because they passed through clinical trials. However, the goals of the trial should be clearly stated and understood before you make the decision. (See the Appendix for more information on clinical trials.)

If something is being tested in a clinical trial, its benefit is still unproven.

42. Does treatment differ if I'm pregnant when diagnosed with ovarian cancer?

Most women who get ovarian cancer do so after menopause. Pregnancy-associated ovarian cancer is a rare, but devastating, diagnosis. It can occur in 1 in 12,000 to 50,000 pregnancies. Often the diagnosis is made surgically, after women present with an abnormal routine ultrasound showing a complex cyst. CT scans are not safe during pregnancy; however, if a complex cyst is found by ultrasound in a pregnant patient, then an MRI may be done.

The first step in management is surgical, as it would be if you were not pregnant. Every attempt should be made at complete surgical staging, which means that an open procedure or laparotomy must be performed.

Unfortunately the decisions are not ones made easily. If you have advanced cancer with spread around the pelvis or abdomen, then your doctors may recommend that the pregnancy be terminated so that the most aggressive treatment can be used to give you the best chance of surviving the cancer. If you are early-staged but considered at a high risk for recurrence, some may advocate delaying treatment until after the first trimester, or even after the birth of your child, whereas others may recommend a more aggressive course. On the other end of the spectrum, you may be considered cured after the affected ovary is removed.

If, whatever the circumstance, you decide to continue with the pregnancy, your doctors must take into account your life first and foremost, all the while minimizing the potential risk to the unborn child.

There's not much information to help guide the postsurgical treatment of ovarian cancer in pregnancy. What we do know is that chemotherapy isn't safe during the first trimester, when all of your baby's organs are forming. However, beyond that, it can be safely administered, although there's always the risk of side effects.

Of the chemotherapy available to treat ovarian cancer, the little data available suggest that cisplatin is safe during pregnancy. Carboplatin may also be used, although the risk for lowering of the platelets (thrombocytopenia) may make cisplatin the better choice. The data on paclitaxel is much less clear, and it's not recommended during pregnancy. In women with early stage disease, the potential benefits of chemotherapy must be weighed against the risks of treatment.

Numerous factors must be taken into account, and you, your family, your oncologist, and your obstetrician must engage in a thorough and honest discussion about the pros and cons of all your options.

43. Is there any role for complementary or alternative therapy?

Alternative therapy (medicines used in lieu of standard medical therapies) and complementary therapy (medicines used in conjunction with standard therapies) include a variety of herbal and food remedies, vitamins and other supplements, and traditional treatments such as acupuncture. Such therapies have become increasingly popular with the general public, and many are based upon traditional healing practices that have hundreds of years of use. Whether they actually work is difficult to know due to the lack of clinical trials available on these types of treatments.

Some alternative therapies are nothing more than scams taking advantage of patients' fears and longings for anything that will make the illness go away. They may do no harm—although some herbal agents can harm you—but they also do no good, so you're spending your money for no good reason. For example, there are data strongly suggesting that the use of antioxidants can actually be harmful during chemotherapy treatment.

Some alternative healing practices also address some of the emotional and physiological problems that accompany cancer treatment, so using them may improve the patient's quality of life, even if it doesn't necessarily stop the cancer itself.

Many people are becoming attracted to alternative philosophies of patient care, particularly east and south Asian methods and homeopathic and naturopathic medical systems. Yet there are so many medicines and therapies touted as the next new treatment for cancer, it's hard to know where to start. For a cancer patient anxious to find an effective treatment—or even a way to deal with unpleasant treatment side effects—the list can be bewildering. A recent study of cancer patients showed that as many of 80% were using or had tried such treatments in conjunction with their standard therapeutic regimens, in the hope of either enhancing the action of the regimen or reducing the side effects caused by it. Unfortunately, a large proportion of the patients in the study were taking these alternative therapies without letting their doctors know and suffering side effects as the therapies interfered with or interacted with the action of chemotherapy drugs—which is why many physicians are wary of alternative medicines. Yet part of the problem is that doctors fail to ask whether their patients are using alternative therapies, and patients don't think to tell them. So the most important point to make in any discussion of alternative therapies is: Make sure your doctor knows about them before you start using them.

Relaxation Therapy

It's safe to assume that therapy aimed at relaxing the mind can have a positive impact on a patient fighting cancer.

Although there isn't much research on the topic of alternative medicine, it's safe to assume that therapy aimed at relaxing the mind can have a positive impact on a patient fighting cancer. Relaxation therapy, including massage, yoga, or tai chi, may provide a benefit to the patient by relieving the psychological stress associated with a cancer diagnosis.

Homeopathic and Naturopathic Medicine

Homeopathic and naturopathic medicines are also examples of complete alternative medical systems. Homeopathic medicine is an unconventional Western system that is based on the principle that "like cures like"; that is, that the same substance that in large doses produces the symptoms of an illness, in very minute doses cures it. Naturopathic medicine views disease as a sign that the processes by which the body naturally heals itself are out of balance and emphasizes health restoration rather than disease treatment. Naturopathic physicians employ an array of healing practices, including diet and clinical nutrition; homeopathy; acupuncture; herbal medicine; hydrotherapy (the use of water in a range of temperatures and methods of applications); spinal and soft-tissue manipulation; physical therapies involving electric currents, ultrasound, and light therapy; therapeutic counseling; and pharmacology. Regarding homeopathic and naturopathic remedies, some physicians may recommend not taking antioxidants while on chemotherapy. This is because, in theory, chemotherapy acts by causing oxidative damage to cancer cells, so antioxidants could work against the activity of chemotherapy. If you're going to use alternative medications while undergoing treatment, it's very important to review them with your oncologist to make sure none of them interferes with standard treatments.

I consulted with an oncologist who specializes in Chinese medicine soon after I began treatment. He made the distinction of two separate phases of complimentary treatment; first, as I had chosen the course of chemotherapy, to get me through the chemo in relatively good condition, and then once the treatment was over, to find ways to strengthen and prevent recurrence. I brought the recommended list of supplements to my oncologist, who reviewed and accepted the supplements I would take to protect my digestive tract, help with nausea, and in general help keep me strong.

The Chinese doctor also talked about my "chi" and how during abdominal surgery, according to Chinese medicine, a lot of "chi" escapes. Thinking about it this way helped me to respect my body and think about building up my life force in general, and not only focusing on the specifics of what foods to eat or not to eat. Fresh air, sunshine, fresh water, good simple food, and conscious exercise (especially the Chinese exercises, such as tai chi and chi gong, although I have preferred yoga) all contribute to the healthy buildup of one's chi.

After my diagnosis, I reconnected with a childhood friend, Carrie Lindia, who is a hands-on healer and practices Reiki. I like the idea of this kind of spiritual, hands-on healing and feel it has had a powerful effect. I've learned to practice it on myself and now, after treatment, I am learning more about it.

Soon after my first chemotherapy, I met a person who would radically change the course of my response to the illness and its treatment. Gene Fairly had been practicing Zen meditation for 25 years when he was diagnosed with a deadly throat cancer. After undergoing unsuccessful, hospitalized treatments of chemotherapy and radiation, he was told that he should undergo a major surgery, which had only a limited chance of success and would result in the loss of his voice. Without this surgery, he was told he faced a prognosis of 3 months to live. He knew instinctively that he would not survive the surgery, and as a producer, editor, translator, and great communicator, he did not want to live without the power to speak.

Within 6 months of up to 6 hours a day of intensive meditation, the mass was gone. Having learned and practiced new ways to harness meditation to heal, he devoted his time after his diagnosis and cure to further developing mind-body meditation techniques and teaching them to others.

When I arrived at Gene's home the first time, I was totally over-whelmed and frightened, by the shock of surgery, the specter of chemotherapy, the fear of death. With his guidance, I learned to meditate to acknowledge and dissolve my fear; to listen to cancer cells; to meditate during chemotherapy to direct the flow of medicine to the tumor sites and to protect the healthy cells; to detoxify my liver and kidneys a few days after chemo was completed; and simply to learn the grace of feeling an inner healing power. I meditated before surgery to ask my cells to be calm and be prepared for the surgeon's work, and to cooperate. I meditated to build red and white blood cells when they were low and to face my worst fears.

One might see meditation as giving a sense of control, and it did provide that. But it also imparted peace and, in peace, there's more room for healing than there is in fear. And I fully believe that the mind "does not rest above the body but is diffused through it."[1] Learning to use the power of the mind for physical, emotional, and spiritual healing affected me in a profound way. Gene always said, "If you meditate, you will change." I knew that to survive this illness, I needed to change.

I also briefly tried acupuncture, which I found soothing but was unable to keep up financially. However, I connected to the acupuncturist when he talked about the fatigue being on a "sub-cellular" level. —Andrea Brown

---

1. Frank, AW. *The Wounded Storyteller: Body, Illness, and Ethics.* Chicago: University of Chicago Press, 1995, p. 2.

WHAT TO DO AFTER TREATMENT IS FINISHED

44. Will the CA-125 reading ever go down to zero?

No, it usually will not go down to zero. During your treatment, we will expect that the CA-125 results will normalize, which in most laboratories is to fall below the level of 35 mg/dL. In most women, this means a fall in their CA-125 to the single digit or teens, but in others it will be slightly higher. As long as these changes stay below 35, there is usually no need to be alarmed. Remember that the CA-125 is only one part of the follow-up. It must be taken into consideration with other factors: how you are feeling, your physical examination, and if necessary, a CT scan.

45. How often should I be examined?

If at the end of your treatment, the cancer can't be detected, either on your physical examination, by CT scan, or by your CA-125 reading, you enter routine follow-up. Most experts agree that being seen every 3 months for the first 2 years is enough. These visits should consist of a physical assessment that includes a pelvic examination and CA-125 test. In most women who have their cancer come back, the recurrence generally appears within this time frame. After 2 years, visits can be extended. If your chemotherapy isn't being administered by your surgeon, we feel it's important to continue to follow up with both your surgeon and medical oncologist at regular intervals.

46. Do I need to have CT scans as part of my regular follow-up?

There is no standard recommendation on the frequency of doing repeat CT scans. If you're doing well at your visits and there doesn't appear to be a concern that your cancer has started to grow again, there's no role for a CT scan. However, if your CA-125 reading starts to rise or goes beyond the normal range or you start to experience vague symptoms, a CT scan may be recommended. In some women, the CA-125 is not a marker of their cancer, or it was normal at the time they were diagnosed. In such situations, more attention needs to be paid to the examination results and your symptoms, but it's reasonable to perform CT scans to reevaluate your disease at more frequent intervals, such as every 3 to 6 months.

47. When can I consider myself cured?

In women who are diagnosed with ovarian cancer and have a complete resection or an optimal debulking of their cancer, chemotherapy is done with the intent to cure. Unfortunately, there's no guarantee that you'll be cured. We do know that 80% of women will initially respond to treatment, but only around 30% will not have their cancer return. In clinical studies, we often use an arbitrary time point to determine "cure," and this is 5 years. Once you get past the 5-year mark, the likelihood of the cancer returning becomes lower and lower, and the chances of your living through the cancer become better and better.

The risk of a second cancer is higher in patients who have already had one type of cancer.

48. Do I still need yearly mammograms?

We always recommend continued health maintenance examinations once patients complete treatment. This is because the risk of a second cancer is higher in patients who have already had one type of cancer. So, yes, you will still need a mammogram. Other health maintenance tests that you and your doctor should discuss are a screening colonoscopy and a bone density test (especially if you had both ovaries removed and are not on estrogen replacement, as there is an increased risk for osteoporosis).

The best intentions of trying to protect your loved ones result in feelings of isolation and loneliness.

49. What do I tell my family?

This is an incredibly personal question, but honesty should be the driving principle. Often, the best intentions of trying to protect your loved ones result in feelings of isolation and loneliness on the patient's part, and a sense of helplessness and distance on the part of those of us who love them. Cancer is not a diagnosis that affects only one person; it will affect everyone around you. Instead of trying to handle it alone, take advantage of the support that is likely to be available from family and friends.

When I first knew the likelihood of my diagnosis, I called my therapist first and told my husband second. I was so afraid to tell him, afraid of hurting him, causing him pain. Also, I did not tell my family until I was absolutely sure of my diagnosis, which really occurred only after surgery. I didn't want to cause unnecessary worry or pain, especially to my parents. However, looking back, I realize that by asking my sister alone, with my husband, to be there during my first surgery, I put an enormous strain on them. I think in retrospect it would have been better all around to speak plainly and have the burden be shared, for there's strength and comfort in sharing. There were times when I spoke very frankly to my family about it, and they were strong enough to hear me.

Every family situation is different, so I think everyone will have a different way of handling it. However, I think that trying to protect others by keeping them in the dark creates emotional distance. There may be times when you need that, and I find now that I no longer report to friends and family every time I have a scan, because we've learned to let go a bit, to trust that everything will be okay, and if it isn't, we know we can deal with it as we have in the past. I don't know how you would tell children, but I'll tell you that the one person who verbally acknowledged my struggle, during my first summer vacation home after diagnosis and treatment, was my young nephew Andrew Roithmayr, age 9. He said that he was so happy that I made it, that I and Lance Armstrong were the only people he knew who had survived cancer. I don't think he knew anybody that had had cancer and didn't survive but, given the fear quotient this disease has, it didn't surprise me that he thought of the worst. What did surprise me was the grace and innocence with which he comforted me.

One thing on which my husband and I have come to agree is to "face the facts." I've always preferred getting results from CT scans directly from the doctor rather than reading them myself, unmediated. The doctor helps to put them in context, and always in the context of a plan. However, when we've been anxious about a CA-125 result, we just bite the bullet and call and find out. Not knowing and maintaining a vague feeling of postponing good or bad news can create more anxiety. So, my natural tendency to want to put my head in the sand has been mitigated by my husband's seeing the need to face things directly. We've learned over the years that although the situation may seem dire, the overall outcome has been good. So, we've learned to trust that we will, with the doctors' and God's help, be able to cope. —Andrea Brown

50. What insurance and financial concerns must I address after my diagnosis?

It is important for you to review your health insurance policy to ensure you are covered for surgery, medical treatment, and, if necessary, second or even third consultations. Navigating the medical system can be both frustrating and time-consuming, so it is worthwhile to seek out financial help, which may be available in the financial services office of your hospital or by speaking directly to a representative of your insurance policy. You will need to know what and where you are covered. If you find a doctor that you feel comfortable with who is not a practicing provider within your insurance plan, make sure you know what, if anything, will be covered by your primary insurance, and what portion of the bills you are likely to be personally responsible for. Your providers should be able to direct you toward the right people to speak with when it comes to billing so you can have some estimate of the charges you may incur from surgery and, if applicable, from chemotherapy.

Insurance is one area in which it's important for you, or for someone helping you, to be an advocate. This means being proactive, informed, and organized. Get a copy (either from the insurance company directly or through your workplace) of your insurance policy's "Certificate of Coverage." Read it. Read the fine print. Know your rights and responsibilities (e.g., when you need to get "precertified" for a hospital procedure). Sometimes your doctor's office staff will deal directly with your insurance company regarding preauthorization, so be sure to communicate with your doctor's staff about this. Obtaining precertification (which most often requires only a timely phone call by you or your doctor) is crucial in getting procedures paid for. Without a "precert" number, a claim may be denied even though your insurance company agrees that the procedure is necessary.

Find out whether you have any options to purchase, through your employer, any more comprehensive coverage. If at all possible, don't allow your payments and therefore your coverage to lapse. Once your coverage has lapsed, your insurance company may qualify you with a "preexisting condition," which may not be covered by new insurance. Once you are uninsured, it can be very difficult to get a preexisting condition covered.

Begin immediately by creating files to keep yourself organized. Some suggestions, depending on your type of insurance coverage, are:

- *Medical bills (different files, such as current and to-be-paid; paid; "in-review"; partially paid; in resubmission; in dispute, appeal, or grievance)*
- *EOBs (explanation of benefits), statements that you receive from your insurance company outlining the expenses paid out by the insurance company for services. Make sure you receive the EOBs so that in case a problem arises, you can see how and when payments were made.*
- *Medical correspondence (different files, for example, correspondence to the insurance company, correspondence with doctors, letters of medical necessity)*
- *In-network referrals and precertification numbers*
- *Out-of-network referrals*
- *Prescriptions and receipts*
- *Disability insurance*
- *Laboratory and test results*

- *Log of doctors' visits*
- *List of all doctors with insurance ID numbers, phone, fax, and address (helpful when requesting referrals)*
- *Correspondence with your employer (regarding sick leave, etc.)*

Keeping paperwork in order and responding to it in a timely and effective manner go a long way toward easing anxiety over the feeling of being overwhelmed that can accompany any serious health issue. Even if you don't have insurance, keeping accurate records can assist you in receiving benefits from governmental and private agencies. You may at times need a lot of patience, fortitude, and perseverance to make the system work for you.

Begin by assuming a good and workable relationship with your insurance company, but be prepared—or have a friend or family member be prepared—to be the "squeaky wheel." Keep a detailed log of any phone calls made to the insurance company and hospital billing department, including the gist of the call, the first and last name of the person with whom you spoke, and the date and time of your call.

Find out whether your plan requires you to stay in network or have the option to go out of network and when you need to get referrals. If your insurance plan requires you to stay in network, begin by working with your primary-care doctor in receiving the referrals you need. Your primary-care doctor can play an important role as helper and advocate even if he or she isn't directly treating you for cancer. The easiest route here is to stay within the network, and your medical billing matters should proceed smoothly. However, be aware that in some circumstances you may be able to receive out-of-network coverage if you can't find the care you need within network. Ask whether the out-of-network doctor can become part of your plan, whether you can be covered for at least some of the fees, and whether the doctor provides any special expertise or service that would qualify for coverage under your plan. This will entail extra advocacy on your (or your helper's) part and on the part of your medical team.

If your insurance plan won't cover a doctor you'd like to see and if you can afford it, consider investing in a consultation. Once you've determined the best course of treatment, the administration of that treatment (such as administration of chemo, blood tests, or CT scans) may be performed routinely, in network.

If you find a procedure or doctor's visit not paid as it should be, resubmit the claim as many times as may be needed. If the bill still isn't paid, ask for a review. (Here, the certificate of coverage and your state insurance department can help you to understand procedures involved in requesting reviews, filing grievances, etc.) Ask your doctor's billing staff to help, and get to know the person handling your bills at your doctor's office.

If you find payment for medicines or procedures denied by the insurance company, find out who exactly is saying no and why. Find out whether your insurance company has assigned you a case worker or medical director, and get their names and contact phone numbers. You have the right to appeal, with the help of your state's insurance commissioner, or to file a grievance if you feel that your case isn't being handled properly. Organizations such as the Patient Advocacy Program, your state's insurance department, and your state's congressmen and senators can help here, too. However, do not allow paperwork to get in the way of your receiving timely care.

If you don't have medical insurance, speak to an oncology social worker from the hospital right away to find out your options. Ask whether you can apply to any state, federal, hospital, or pharmaceutical company programs for financial aid or discount. The federal Hill-Burton Program helps certain hospitals and facilities to provide free or low-cost services. Ask your caseworker whether your facility falls within these guidelines and can offer you assistance. If you're a veteran, you may qualify for special assistance. Also, call the American Cancer Society and Cancer Care for help in finding out about financial assistance (e.g., Medicaid, Social Security) for which you may qualify. Above all, have faith that help will be provided, and focus on the immediate need of getting the best health care you can.

If you are denied treatment, contact the American Cancer Society, Cancer Care, and the Patient Advocacy Foundation, and call your state bar association to find out whether any program provides free legal counsel to cancer patients with treatment-denial problems.

Go over medical bills as you receive them, and make sure that you understand them. If need be, go in and speak to someone in the billing department if you have any questions. Sometimes, speaking to someone in person, rather than over the phone, is more effective. If your insurance company is slow in paying your bills and you begin receiving collection notices, try to work together with the hospital billing department and insurance company in resolving such matters. A hospital social worker or case worker can help here, too.

Getting involved in billing and insurance matters can be very taxing and emotional. I learned to limit my time dealing with insurance matters to two hours a day, and I hope that you will not need anywhere near that time. Otherwise—and I've heard this from others—the insurance-billing behemoth can consume you. Be practical and get a little done each day rather than trying to solve all the issues in one go. I also tried to maintain a positive attitude when speaking with the claims department workers and even began ringing a Tibetan bell (ever so softly) at the beginning of each billing conversation to help smooth the way! This worked even better than a tranquilizer for me. Working on these matters can become very stressful and consuming, and it either can serve as a potent and concrete reminder of your health situation or as an unhealthy outlet for anger and frustration. So, keep up your records as best you can, work on problems in a paced and consistent manner, and learn when to stop and not get stressed out. —Andrea Brown

PART FOUR

Coping with Treatment-Related Side Effects

Should I take special precautions while on chemotherapy?

What kind of diet should I follow while on treatment? What about after treatment?

Will I be able to tolerate treatment if I am older?

More...

51. Should I take special precautions while on chemotherapy?

Many people are under the impression that chemotherapy will require them to live in their homes unable to eat fresh fruit, enjoy flowers, other people, the movies, or even their own children or grandchildren. Yes, chemotherapy requires some diligence in terms of monitoring your own temperature if you feel warm or suspect a fever, but a woman doesn't need to change her entire life and surroundings due to the type of chemotherapy we use for ovarian cancer. The reason that many of these precautions are taken is to avoid any risk of infection when you are most vulnerable after chemotherapy, which is when your white counts decrease (called neutropenia) and you are prone to develop infections and fever. This time at risk is variable depending on what cancer you have and the regimen being used to treat it. People undergoing treatment for leukemia or who have had a bone marrow transplant are most at risk because the periods of neutropenia are very long. Fortunately, for women being treated for ovarian cancer this time is not long-lasting; in general it lasts less than a week. Therefore, they do not need to undergo this degree of protection.

A woman doesn't need to change her entire life and surroundings due to the type of chemotherapy we use for ovarian cancer.

52. What kind of diet should I follow while on treatment? What about after treatment?

There's a substantial amount of information about diet and its role in healing and cancer therapy. Unfortunately, none of it has been studied to any great degree, and there aren't a lot of data to help guide us in the role of diet in cancer care. A lot of patients have heard about avoiding refined sugar or white flour, because these may contribute to cancer. The bottom line is that no studies have linked diet to chemotherapy response or to a risk of recurrence. It is probably best to eat a variety of foods in moderation and to follow a heart-healthy diet. After all, the cancer does not define the patient. You are still the same person you were before cancer, at risk for heart disease and high blood pressure. Treat your body well by eating a balanced diet and allow yourself the time to heal.

I found the best diet that worked for me was a diet high in fiber. Other than that, drinking plenty of fluids, such as water, juices, and limited amounts of decaffeinated coffee and teas, helps me get through treatments. —Phyllis Hames

53. Will I be able to tolerate treatment if I am older?

Treating older patients (beyond age 60) is another evolving area of study. Earlier studies suggested that age was an important factor in the prognosis for women suffering from ovarian cancer and that older women did not do as well as younger women. This theory has been subjected to more debate as we have recognized an important bias: Older patients generally are not given the same treatment options as those offered to younger patients. In fact, older women tolerate chemotherapy as well as do younger women, and the more important factor to consider is not age but the activity you're able to perform on a daily basis (your **performance status**). It is well recognized that a sicker patient who requires 24-hour home care and cannot walk without assistance will fare worse with chemotherapy than will a healthier patient, regardless of age.

Older women tolerate chemotherapy as well as do younger women.

Performance status

A numerical description of how a person is doing in her normal day-to-day life and whether her cancer is impacting her ability to live normally.

Having said this, it may be wise to tailor therapy for women past the age of 70 and for those in specific situations, such as women with an underlying neuropathy from diabetes or other causes or those having a baseline hearing loss.

54. Should I be taking any special vitamins?

Your doctor may recommend a multivitamin a day. Anything more than that is generally not necessary. As exists for dietary advice, a lot of information has been circulated regarding vitamin supplementation to help the immune system and even about the use of homeopathic remedies, such as coral calcium and shark cartilage. Unfortunately, there aren't a lot of data to tell whether these homeopathic remedies or vitamin supplements are actually helping you. The major goal is to stay away from things that could eventually hurt you, and you need to discuss and review fully with your doctor all nontraditional medications before you start taking them. As was discussed earlier, taking antioxidants such as vitamin E and vitamin C may be a bad thing during chemotherapy.

55. What's a growth factor? When would I need it?

Growth factors are drugs that stimulate the bone marrow to recover after chemotherapy. They are available to help stimulate your red blood cells and white blood cells.

Erythropoietin is a hormone that stimulates your body to release red blood cells. Two drugs are available that essentially act like erythropoietin, epoetin alfa (aka Procrit) and darbepoetin alfa (aka Aranesp). Both are used to treat or prevent chemotherapy-induced anemia. A growth factor is usually recommended by your doctor if your hemoglobin falls below a certain level. For it to work, your doctor would need to check your iron levels to make sure you do not have an alternative reason to be anemic. Keeping you from becoming anemic has been shown to improve the way you feel during chemotherapy and also helps decrease the chances you will need a blood transfusion.

Both agents are given as an injection into your skin (subcutaneously). The difference between the two agents is how long they are active in your body. Epoetin alfa has to be used either three times a week or weekly (I use it weekly) because it does not stick around any longer than 7 days. Darbepoetin alfa is designed to stick around longer and therefore can be used every 2 weeks. Studies have shown they are equally effective.

Filgrastim (Neupogen) and pegfilgrastim (Neulasta) are both used to treat low white blood cell counts from chemotherapy. If your doctor thinks you're at a high risk for this complication, it may be recommended to you as a protective move. Otherwise, you may not need it and it would be used only if you had experienced a problem with your counts, such as fevers or even infections due to low blood counts (neutropenic fever), which may require you to be hospitalized. The use of these drugs can shorten the time your white blood cell counts are low. A low white blood cell count is a risk for getting an infection, which can be very serious.

These drugs also allow you to be treated on schedule, without delays or disruption, so you can complete treatment as anticipated. Filgrastim requires a daily injection into your skin, which usually begins the day after treatment and continues for 3–5 days. Pegfilgrastim stays in your system longer (about 2 weeks), so it needs to be administered only once between chemotherapy sessions.

56. How do you control nausea? What are the different medicines used?

As stated earlier, nausea is a common side effect of the chemotherapy used to treat ovarian cancer, and in some women can be a very significant side effect. Fortunately, we have strong anti-nausea medications that can specifically treat and even prevent nausea.

Ondansetron (Zofran) and granisetron (Kytril) are very potent anti-nausea drugs. They work by blocking specific pathways for nausea that are triggered by chemotherapy and work through the nervous system protein serotonin. They are available in pill form and as an injection. One dose is administered before chemotherapy treatment and then is taken by mouth at home, usually for 3 days after chemotherapy, when you're at most risk for chemotherapy-induced nausea and vomiting. A newer agent in this class, palonosetron (Aloxi), may be recommended if the others do not work. This is available only as an injection and is useful only to prevent, not to treat, nausea.

Aprepitant (Emend) is a new drug approved in 2005 for the prevention of nausea associated with chemotherapy. It also works on the nervous system, but blocks neurokinin 1 (NK1), a protein found in the brain that causes vomiting. It is taken 1 hour before chemotherapy and then again in the morning for the next 2 days. It's used in addition to other anti-nausea drugs, such as ondansetron or granisetron.

If you are going to be treated with cisplatin, then there is a risk that you may experience nausea for more than 3 days after treatment. These delayed side effects from chemotherapy are treated with steroids—most commonly dexamethasone (Decadron). These are usually taken once or twice daily and then doses are reduced over the next 4 or 5 days, called a steroid taper.

Benzodiazepines like lorazepam (Ativan) also are used to treat nausea and vomiting, in addition to being used to treat nervousness and anxiety.

Finally, prochlorperazine (Compazine) is prescribed as a general anti-vomiting drug. It is available as a pill or as a suppository, and can be used for nausea and vomiting that occurs at any point during treatment for cancer. Some women don't particularly like it due to some of its side effects like nervousness or jitteriness.

It's very important that your doctor be aware of how you are doing before, during, and after chemotherapy treatments. Often, with adjustments in treatment or in the medications used, nausea can be very well controlled and need not be a significant problem.

57. What can I do about the chemotherapy-related numbness and tingling?

During treatment, you will be asked about problems with numbness or tingling (neuropathy). These can occur due to the taxanes or to cisplatin. Make sure your doctor knows if this develops and, more importantly, make sure it is being followed on treatment because it can get progressively worse. If not addressed early on, it can get so bad that it may affect your ability to do fine movements, such as buttoning your blouse, turning a door knob, or operating a can opener.

If symptoms develop, there are medications that you can take to help prevent it from getting worse, and you should discuss them with your doctor. Some patients benefit from taking a vitamin called glutamine, available at most natural food stores or vitamin shops. Others get relief from the pain associated with neuropathy with the use of gabapentin (Neurontin). If your symptoms worsen, your doctor may manage them by reducing the dose of paclitaxel or switching to another drug altogether, docetaxel, which has less risk of causing neuropathy. One study done in Europe showed that docetaxel with carboplatin was as effective as paclitaxel with carboplatin, so you should not worry about such a change decreasing your chances of beating ovarian cancer.

58. Can I work while receiving treatment?

Although the treatment for ovarian cancer is very tolerable, it is generally a good idea to take some time off work when you start treatment, particularly if you choose to go through intraperitoneal (IP) treatment. IP therapy is a complicated process and may require you to be hospitalized for a portion of treatment.

For those patients on intravenous chemotherapy, some may be relatively unaffected by their treatment and will be able to work while on therapy, but others will find that they do

It is generally a good idea to take some time off work when you start treatment, particularly if you choose to go through intraperitoneal (IP) treatment.

not have the energy to devote to both a job and to chemotherapy.

Remember that although most treatments are now done as outpatient procedures, they still require a lot of time. Carboplatin and paclitaxel, for example, can take 6 hours from start to finish. This is why many women often choose to go on disability while on chemotherapy and concentrate on getting better so that they are more able to return to work in a productive capacity.

I worked part-time during most of my treatments, but was fortunate enough to have a very flexible work schedule that could be adjusted at any time. There were days when sudden sickness came on and I had to cancel work. I would say that everyone is different, and it depends on the kind of work you do and what kind of treatment you're on. —Phyllis Hames

I was able to work, albeit at reduced hours, while getting treatment and felt it was "good for my head." But I think it depends a lot on the kind of work you do. This is partly due to infection risks: My cousin, who was a nursery school teacher, was advised against working because of it, and I had to be careful around my college students. I'd advise anyone who works around lots of people to carry Purell around with them and use it frequently.

But the other thing that's hard about working is that you lose a lot of control over your schedule when in treatment. On Carbo/Taxol I was able to plan my treatment and work schedule around the day 3–5 bone pain once I knew to expect it. But I couldn't control for treatment delays when my cell counts were too low, which meant having to go for more frequent blood tests and not being sure when my next treatment would be. On Carbo/Gemzar I didn't have the bone pain but had more cell-count delays, and also needed to get a platelet transfusion a couple of times. So there's always a need for last minute rearrangements, and I think the ability to work hinges on being able to arrange for flexible hours and, if possible, working at least some of the time from home. I was fortunate that I was able to arrange this. With both regimens it also helped a lot that I have a private office at work where I could lie down and nap if I needed to. —Marsha Posusney

59. Will I still be able to care for my kids while receiving chemotherapy? What about my pets?

You should be able to carry out most normal activities even while on chemotherapy. You should not put aside your goals and needs. In fact, most studies show that some people feel better on treatment than they did when they were diagnosed. You need not sequester yourself from your family or your pets while receiving treatment. You may be more tired, particularly as you near completion of your treatment, and may need some help in taking care of your pets or home responsibilities. However, with a little help from your friends and family, you should be able to continue your normal routines. This means, however, that you must accept help when it's offered. Many people politely refuse an offer from a friend or family member, thinking they don't want to burden others with their illness, but this habit only makes your difficult task of recovery more difficult than it needs to be. If your family and friends want to help, let them!

Most studies show that some people feel better on treatment than they did when they were diagnosed.

60. Can I still have sex even while I'm in treatment?

A woman's vagina can thin considerably and be prone to irritation due to a lack of estrogen after the ovaries are removed. This can make intercourse uncomfortable. Even more commonly, many women suffer a loss of sexual interest from the psychological impact of being diagnosed with ovarian cancer, surgical debulking, and the physical manifestations of undergoing chemotherapy, most notably the loss of hair. All of these factors may work together to help dampen any interest in sex. However, this does not have to be the case. With a trusting partner and patience, as women come to accept their diagnosis and the treatments at hand, it is more common for women to rediscover themselves as sexual persons and, together with a patient and understanding partner, ultimately recover their sexuality. Your doctor can help in this area, but it requires an open and honest discussion about sexuality. Medication, such as vaginal estrogen in low doses, vaginal dilators, and lubrication aids, are available to help you maintain or rediscover a satisfying sexual life.

The Vagifem (the low-dose estrogen pill you insert into your vagina on a regular basis) has helped a lot, although I did not begin this treatment until after chemo treatment was done. I was very concerned about "vaginal atrophy," whereby the tissues thin out and become very easily chafed. I also found that using a really mild soap (for instance, Dove) to clean myself was not irritating. And then there are such products as Replens, which help to keep your vagina moisturized, and such lubricants as AstroGlide for sexual intercourse. My husband and I continued to have a sex life during my treatment, but there were periods in which, owing to physical and emotional side effects of things (surgery, examinations, chemo, and lack of estrogen), I didn't feel much like having sex.

At one point I did ask for a vaginal dilator, which is basically a set of smaller and larger tube-shaped items to give the vagina ever more strenuous "work-outs." I never even opened the box, although I always meant to. I've had to work at keeping up an active sex life, and my husband has been a help here, being very gentle and patient. I imagined myself using a dildo and vibrator to practice, but I haven't gotten there yet, although it's probably a good idea. Talking to a therapist or sharing your feelings in an all-women group can really help here, too.

The lessening of hormones and the trauma of surgery—and even examinations—sometimes made sex seem like the last thing on my mind. However, I found that with practice, communication, a patient husband, some good lubrication, intravaginal estrogen, some sex toys, and some humor, I have been able to resume a relatively active sex life.

I think pampering yourself can go a long way here, too. Treating yourself to a nice long bubble bath, a massage by a professional or just a friend, an evening polishing and buffing, and keeping your skin soft with moisturizers can go a long way to continue feeling soft and feminine. During chemo is an especially important time to love yourself and your body, and taking the time to do these gentle activities for yourself can be rewarding. —Andrea Brown

I avoided intercourse because I'm prone to bladder infections from it, and also to minor lacerations even when using lubricant. But (Bill Clinton's word games notwithstanding) there are other satisfying forms of sex that don't risk infection. —Marsha Posusney

61. Taking my ovaries has suddenly made me have hot flashes. Is this menopause? What can I do for relief?

Removal of the ovaries will obviously result in a significant decrease of estrogen and progesterone from the circulation. A consequence of that is menopause, which sometimes may be symptomatic; patients may have hot flashes, night sweats, mood changes, and vaginal discomfort with burning and painful intercourse. The treatment of symptomatic menopause is best achieved with hormone replacement therapy. Hormone replacement therapy is usually given as a tablet, a skin patch, or a local vaginal cream or vaginal tablet, depending on the symptoms and the area that needs to be treated.

Patients who have had a total hysterectomy and who need hormone replacement therapy usually require estrogen only. However, patients who still have a uterus must take both estrogen and progesterone, because taking unopposed estrogen will increase the likelihood of uterine and endometrial malignancy.

Hormone replacement therapy is usually safe in the setting of ovarian carcinoma; however, it should be reserved for patients who have significant menopause-related symptoms.

The lowest dose of estrogen and the shortest duration needed to help alleviate the symptoms should be used, because long-term use of hormone replacement therapy may be associated with side effects such as increased risk of breast cancer or venous thromboembolism. The decision of whether to take hormone replacement therapy will depend on a thorough discussion with your gynecologic oncologist or medical oncologist; however, if your symptoms are severe, a low-dose hormone replacement therapy may significantly improve the symptoms and improve your quality of life.

62. Is depression common after treatment?

Yes, depression is a common experience for women with ovarian cancer. Once a woman is diagnosed, she may work through a whole gamut of emotions like terror, fear, anxiety, and worry. However, as many women begin therapy, a sense of resolve and a determination to do whatever is necessary to beat the cancer soon sets in. Yet, as much as a woman looks forward to completing treatment, it is not uncommon for many to feel a sense of depression after treatment has been completed. It is often due to a sense of anxiety that nothing is being done once treatment is over (entering the "watchful waiting" period), and with that, a loss of control over what the future may hold. Many women can work through this with the passage of time, as they become more used to the frequent schedule of follow-up visits. But for some, the end of therapy brings about a sense of sadness and a sometimes overwhelming fear, which can be quite debilitating. If this appears to be occurring, it is very important to discuss such concerns with your physician. After all, no woman diagnosed with ovarian cancer should live the rest of her life paralyzed by fear or depression over what may be.

No woman diagnosed with ovarian cancer should live the rest of her life paralyzed by fear or depression.

63. When will my hair grow back?

Once you complete treatment with paclitaxel, your hair should start growing back, but certainly you should have noticeable hair growth within 3 months of stopping treatment. It may take 6 months, or even longer, to have shoulder-length hair. Do not be surprised or shocked if your hair grows back different in texture, style, or color. It may begin as gray or even white, and in more than a few women, it has come back curly. As you get farther out from treatment, your hair should resume its normal appearance as it was before you started therapy. But patience will be necessary before you get to that point.

Do not be surprised or shocked if your hair grows back different in texture, style, or color.

64. Does chemotherapy affect your memory?

A common complaint in women being treated with chemotherapy is a decrease in memory, sometimes called "chemobrain." They complain of an inability to retain short-term memories, like what they just talked about with friends or where they put their keys. These problems can impact on their daily lives, especially if they take care of a household or are doing a mentally demanding task. Still, it is important to realize that these issues are poorly understood, and chemotherapy-induced changes in memory have not been identified in recent studies.

65. Will I ever enjoy my own life again?

There is no question that being diagnosed with ovarian cancer will change your life. But this does not mean it must be for the worse. Many women find a renewed sense of spirituality after their diagnosis. In addition, it is not uncommon for a life-threatening diagnosis to shock someone into realizing the important things in life. In this way, being diagnosed with cancer can paradoxically improve your life by reminding you how important you are to you and what an important goal your personal happiness is.

Many women find a renewed sense of spirituality after their diagnosis.

Having said this, it is also common for women to suffer from anxiety over what the future may hold. However, even in this case, time is the best medicine. As you get farther and farther out from treatment, the follow-ups, the blood tests, and the radiology exams become routine, and you will be able to find a balance between the "worry" and the "rest of your life" that works best for you.

There are many layers to the cancer experience, and in meditation group we talked about not getting "cancer mind." I would describe cancer mind as forming an attachment to the disease or identifying yourself too closely with it. Yes, I'm sure there is a mind–body connection and, after a cancer diagnosis, nothing is really ever the same. There's a loss of innocence, a loss of any sense of immortality you may have been able to hold onto from childhood. And then there is hair loss, and maybe some weight loss, and possibly fertility and job loss—there's a lot to cope with emotionally.

These losses didn't really begin to hit me for some time after treatment, as I was so focused on fighting the disease and coping with the chemo that I couldn't really process much else. In this sense, too, I think it can hit loved ones even harder, as they are helpless to do anything, although they may be able to take in the psychological impact earlier. When it did finally hit me, I found it difficult but necessary to speak frankly with my partner about my fears. I was trying to protect him but, when I did that, I found that it really created distance between us.

That being said, I also think it's of immense importance to attend a group, because I think you can wear out your friends and family with talking about cancer, whereas in a group you can be really free to speak as much as you need to. The most valuable things I gained from attending groups were a sense of not being alone and meeting two women who became close friends. These friendships are very important to me, because we understand each other so much and can share, listen, and gripe without feeling a need to explain or excuse ourselves.

I think the fear and the frustration that come with your diagnosis and its aftereffects can really inhibit your ability to forget yourself and enjoy life. For me, beginning meditation was the difference between having some psychological freedom and ease and feeling trapped in fear. I cannot emphasize enough the difference it made for me. In it, I was able to find some peace in the midst of the life-threatening struggle. I worked one-on-one with my beloved teacher, the late Gene Fairly, who had coped with a cancer diagnosis himself, in developing a mind–body visualization-based meditation, and I worked within a group. Writing about the experience has reminded me how crucial this was to my well-being, and I am renewing my commitment to meditation. Gene would always say, "If you meditate, you will change." That's true, and you may find more strength of spirit than you were aware you had.

I've learned that I can forget I have cancer when I immerse myself in activities outside my head, which for me is through creative endeavor. I have always made it a goal to keep up with my creative activities during treatment, and that has given me something on which to focus outside the health realm. Sometimes, my entire life in every sense was consumed by the illness. I had to pray a lot, and at turns I asked for peace, strength, courage, forgiveness, and guidance. —Andrea Brown

On carboplatin and paclitaxel I was able to exercise a bit (walking) even during treatment, and return to other activities gradually afterwards. It took about a month after the cycle ended for me to be back to prior exercise levels. On Carbo/Gemzar my energy levels improved after I started getting Aranesp; the weather hasn't cooperated much with my outdoor exercise plans, but I will return to indoor ice skating tomorrow (one week after end of last cycle).

You can enjoy life even during treatment—we planned short trips to local resorts and just enjoyed the scenery if I was too tired for anything else. I also highly recommend "shopping therapy." Even a new pair of fun socks can be a big boost to sagging spirits. —Marsha Posusney

PART FIVE

Symptom Management

How does ovarian cancer cause abdominal pain?

What can I do for constipation?

How do I manage pain?

More...

66. How does ovarian cancer cause abdominal pain?

Ovarian cancer may cause abdominal or pelvic pain for a variety of reasons. The pain may be related to a large ovarian mass that is pulling on the ligaments inside you or sometimes the mass can twist (torsion) and that will cause severe pain. The other causes of pain or pressure may be related to the ovarian tumor; to an abdominal tumor pressing on other organs such as the bladder, the rectum, or the intestine; or to internal bleeding related to the tumor. Obviously, if there is a large volume of tumor inside the abdomen with ascites (fluid) or bulky upper abdominal disease, this may cause pressure on the intestines or stomach and will cause pain and discomfort. The symptoms of ovarian cancer may be subtle and mild; however, any change in abdominal symptoms or bloating or indigestion should be reported to your physician promptly.

If you develop abdominal pain, it's very important that you immediately consult with your physician or seek care in an emergency room to find a reason for your pain and specifically to rule out an intestinal obstruction. The evaluation will require a physical examination and imaging studies, usually abdominal x-rays and a CT scan of your abdomen and pelvis. Intestinal obstruction, a very common complication of advanced or recurrent ovarian cancer, may require surgery.

Patient-controlled analgesia (PCA)

A method of providing pain medication through the vein that allows direct control over the amount required to make one comfortable.

If your physician believes that you might have an obstruction, you will have to go to the hospital. Your doctor may recommend surgery to correct the obstruction. If your pain is severe, you may require morphine or another type of narcotic, which may be offered to you as an infusion pump that allows you to control directly the amount of pain medication you get (**patient-controlled analgesia**).

It's important to realize that abdominal pain does not automatically mean that you have an obstruction. There are other possible causes for pain, and most of them can be managed without having to admit you to the hospital. Some common causes are constipation, kidney stones, or a urinary tract infection. However, an obstruction may become an emergency, and then it requires immediate evaluation to rule it out.

67. What can I do for constipation?

Constipation is a very common complaint for women with ovarian cancer. It is typically present at diagnosis and can persist throughout treatments and recurrence. Because ovarian cancer tends to grow along the surface of your bowels, the normal function of the bowels is affected, which results in constipation. You may require the use of laxatives and stool softeners, such as senna and Colace. If constipation is related to pain medications or progression of your cancer, these may not work well enough. Your doctor may recommend other medications, including lactulose, magnesium citrate, and enemas, to help with bowel movements.

Sometimes chemotherapy treatments can cause constipation, and I try to follow a high fiber diet, which works for me. You could try over-the-counter fiber supplements, which have helped. There are medications that can help, such as stool softeners (Colace) and senna-based medicines (Senokot) which can also help. You should talk with your chemotherapy nurse and your doctor about it before it gets worse. They can help you find the best solution. —ZoeAnn King

68. How do I manage pain?

A primary goal of anyone involved in the treatment of cancer patients is to alleviate pain. It is always important for your doctor to perform a history of the pain, exam, and diagnostic studies to determine the source of your pain. If it is related to your cancer, often it is relieved as the cancer shrinks with chemotherapy. However, the use of narcotics is often essential to help with pain. If your doctor is unsure how to dose your pain medication or if the pain is not being controlled accurately, there are now specialists in pain management whom you can see. If the pain is found to be due to a specific site of cancer that is pressing on nerves, your doctor may even recommend radiation to help relieve the pain.

69. Will the fatigue end after treatment? What can I do for it?

Fatigue is a common side effect of chemotherapy, drug therapy, and the cancer itself. Many women find their own personal way of coping with it. If you are found to be anemic, often using medications like epogen (Procrit) will help by increasing your red cell count. If you are on chemotherapy, drinking fluids may help by preventing dehydration. Try not to restrict yourself solely to water; use fluids rich in metabolites to replenish important electrolytes that may be lost as your body copes with the chemotherapy. Fatigue may also be a side effect of medications, like the anti-nausea agents and pain medications. If this is happening to you, talk to your doctor about alternatives that may be available but not cause as much tiredness. Finally, try your best to stay active, even though it may be difficult at first. You may find it becomes easier with time.

70. How do I manage my emotions?

Find an outlet for your emotions.

Perhaps one of the most important messages we can provide is to find an outlet for your emotions. It is not good to keep them inside, because those feelings will find some way of coming to the surface. Yes, you must bring your own personal strength to the treatments for cancer, but you don't have to be a superhero. Accept your limitations, cry when you need to, and ask for help when you cannot do it alone. Remember that women before you have walked the same road, and as such, consider yourself part of an exclusive club that you never imagined you'd join. But you are a part of a community of women with and survivors of ovarian cancer. If help is needed, all you must do is reach out.

Many emotions surface with a diagnosis of ovarian cancer: anxiety, depression, sadness, fear, and self-pity. . . . All of these emotions are valid; your life has just been turned upside down. I believe that you as the patient have the responsibility to set the tone for your family and treatment team. The diagnosis of ovarian cancer is frightening, but it does not mean your life is over—just changed. If you can set a positive tone, then everyone can feel right in line with you. This will make the treatment process easier on everyone. You may realize it is not an easy task and that you need help. There are a variety of resources for support from support groups you could join, or speaking with a social worker or counselor. If you're having trouble keeping your emotions in control, then I urge you to speak with your doctor. He/she may recommend medication to help you get back on track. —ZoeAnn King

PART SIX

Relapse

How can my ovarian cancer come back if my ovaries have already been removed?

What happens if the cancer comes back?

How do you make a diagnosis of recurrence?

More...

71. How can my ovarian cancer come back if my ovaries have already been removed?

Ovarian cancer cells can escape outside the ovary and be present in many parts of the pelvic and abdominal cavity, particularly in the lining of the peritoneum. They can hide in lymph nodes in any part of your body, or even can show up as microscopic cells in your lung, liver, bone, or brain. Removal of the ovaries will ensure that the original site of cancer is removed, but it does not guarantee that the cancer will not show up elsewhere in your body.

Removal of the ovaries will ensure that the original site of cancer is removed, but it does not guarantee that the cancer will not show up elsewhere in your body.

At the time of diagnosis, you may have a small but undetectable volume of cancer cells floating throughout your peritoneum and your entire body; if not treated, these cells may grow and eventually present as a tumor recurrence. This is why most patients with ovarian cancer should receive postsurgical (or adjuvant) chemotherapy. It's a way to secure the destruction of any potential "microscopic metastasis" that may have escaped the ovaries.

72. What happens if the cancer comes back?

If ovarian cancer recurs, your treatment will depend on where the cancer is found and the length of the interval away from chemotherapy (also known as the **treatment-free interval**, or TFI). The TFI is usually measured from the date of the last chemotherapy treatment after your initial surgery to the date of recurrence. In general, if your cancer comes back and requires treatment with another round of chemotherapy within 6 months (after you completed the prior treatment), it's considered unlikely to respond to another round of platinum-based chemotherapy, sometimes referred to as platinum resistance. Your oncologist will generally offer you other chemotherapy drugs that work in a different way, so-called **second-line chemotherapy**. Patients whose disease returns after a short time will generally not do as well as those who have a recurrence after a year or more. If ovarian cancer recurs more than 6 months after you complete your chemotherapy,

Treatment-free interval

The time between the end of one chemotherapy regimen and initiation of a subsequent therapy for recurrent disease.

Second-line chemotherapy

Chemotherapy given during recurrence.

treatment will be based on where the cancer has reappeared and on your TFI. Occasionally, recurrent ovarian cancer can be cured with a combination of multimodality treatment that involves surgery, chemotherapy, and even radiation.

It is important to remember when you have a recurrence that you can re-enter treatment. There are many treatment options available to you. My cancer recurred about four years ago. In that time, I have had a number of different treatments, and more are available that I have not yet tried. You always have choices. You and your doctor must make the decisions together and do what is best for you. —ZoeAnn King

73. How do you make a diagnosis of recurrence?

As mentioned earlier, women in follow-up for ovarian cancer are usually seen every 3 to 4 months and followed by physical examination and CA-125. If your cancer recurs, you will usually present with symptoms, such as abdominal swelling, increased tiredness, inability to eat, or changes in your bowel function. Sometimes they will be similar to how you originally presented. If there is a clinical suspicion of disease recurrence, a CA-125 and imaging are very important parts of the work-up. The CA-125 measure should be interpreted as a guide that you and your physician can use to monitor the activity of your cancer. The absolute number is not as important as how rapidly it's changing. Studies now show that the rate at which the CA-125 measurement doubles above normal is an important predictor of disease growth.

A rising CA-125 can be the first sign of a recurrence. Often, it precedes the cancer's showing up on a CT scan by 2 to 3 months or even longer. A recent small study from Johns Hopkins suggested that even changes within the normal range of the CA-125 measure were predictive of recurrent disease. Changes of 50% to 100% of the smallest value were a strong predictor of recurrent disease. The situation in which the

CA-125 reading is elevated without any other evidence of cancer is called a **serological relapse**. If you have no symptoms of recurrence outside of the CA-125, then you and your oncologist need to determine what treatment is best for you. Currently there is no real standard of how to treat women who have a serological relapse—some women proceed with chemotherapy to get to a normal CA-125 again, whereas others undergo close observation with monthly serum CA-125s or treatment using anti-estrogen medications such as tamoxifen or letrozole (see **Table 5**). Repeat CT scans at more regular intervals (e.g., every 6 to 8 weeks) may also be performed to make sure that the cancer is not starting to grow. An ongoing clinical trial being conducted in Europe is comparing immediate versus delayed chemotherapy for treating serological relapse. The results of this trial will help us to decide how best to treat women with a rising CA-125 but no other evidence of recurrent disease.

Table 5   Hormonal agents that may be used in the treatment of ovarian cancer

Estrogen blockers block estrogen stimulation on tumor cells.
 • Tamoxifen

Aromatase inhibitors block a protein called aromatase, which converts adrenal hormones (also known as androgens) to estrogens; ultimately leads to estrogen blockade at the tumor cell.
 • Anastrazole
 • Letrozole
 • Exemestane

Gonadotropic-releasing hormone agonists work in the brain on the pituitary gland and cause an initial rise in sex-related hormones—testosterone in men and estradiol in women—but with more frequent administration cause a reduction of circulating hormone levels.
 • Leuprolide acetate

If the disease can be detected by imaging techniques (CT scan, MRI scan, or even PET scan) most oncologists will recommend treatment. The type of treatment will depend on several factors: whether your symptoms are related to the cancer, how much cancer is present, the interval between the end of your treatment and the discovery of the recurrent tumor, and how you're feeling overall. However, in regard to recurrent cancer, you should explore all therapeutic options. They could include the possibility of a second operation to resect (remove) the recurrent cancer, chemotherapy, and perhaps even the use of radiation.

74. How do you make a decision on who could benefit from surgery for recurrent disease?

This is a very important question because new and emerging data suggest that a large percentage of patients with recurrent ovarian carcinoma may benefit from reoperation and removal of this tumor prior to more treatment with chemotherapy or even radiation therapy. The choice of women for a "secondary cytoreduction" or re-operation to remove recurrent cancer depends on the following selection criteria:

- Your disease-free interval; in other words, how many months since stopping the first treatment you have been without evidence of disease before this recurrence was identified
- Whether the recurrence involves a single site or multiple sites in the body
- Whether there is disease throughout your abdomen or pelvis (also called carcinomatosis)

In general, patients must be medically fit to undergo surgery and without an obvious contraindication to a laparotomy, which is an open procedure in the abdomen or pelvis. At Memorial Sloan-Kettering Cancer Center, the general selection criteria to offer secondary cytoreduction for recurrent ovarian carcinoma include patients with a single site of recurrence that has occurred at least 6 months since the completion of chemotherapy—in other words, a disease-free interval of at least 6 months. In fact, the longer the disease-free interval, the better the outcome is for these patients. This single site of recurrence may be in the pelvis or the abdomen or sometimes the liver or the lung. Usually, patients who have a single site of recurrent ovarian carcinoma may benefit from secondary cytoreductive surgery where this tumor is removed, particularly if the disease-free interval is long.

Patients who have multiple sites of recurrences but no obvious carcinomatosis may also benefit from secondary cytoreduction, particularly if the disease-free interval is greater than one year. Patients who have carcinomatosis and large ascites are the least likely to benefit from secondary reoperation; however, there may be a role in highly selected patients: those women with carcinomatosis but with a disease-free interval of more than 30 months after their completion of primary chemotherapy.

In summary, patients who have recurrent ovarian carcinoma may benefit significantly from discussing whether a secondary operation may be of benefit in their disease. This discussion is best held with a gynecologic oncologist. As our understanding of the management of recurrent ovarian carcinoma improves, more and more patients may benefit from reoperation for recurrent disease, particularly if the disease-free interval is greater than one year and the recurrence is isolated to a single site or to a few sites without evidence of carcinomatosis.

75. If the cancer comes back, can I still be cured?

Recurrences will happen to many women with ovarian cancer.

Recurrences will happen to many women with ovarian cancer, particularly if they originally were found to have stage III or stage IV disease, and for the majority of women who recur, cure is not a realistic goal. However, recurrence does not equal terminal disease. On the contrary, with the many treatment options available to women with ovarian cancer, one can expect to survive the recurrence and experience a second or greater remission or to live with recurrent ovarian cancer as a chronic medical condition.

Rarely, a patient may be found to have recurrence in only one area within the pelvis. In this kind of situation, using a combination of surgery, chemotherapy, and radiation, oncologists can once again treat the disease with the hope of a long remission.

In those patients whose tumor recurs and is found in multiple areas of their abdomen or pelvis (or both) or whose disease has traveled to their lungs, liver, or elsewhere, the cancer is not curable. There is effective treatment that may be able to reduce the volume of disease and even put your disease back into remission. However, a remission does not last for long, and you will likely be in and out of treatment for the rest of your life.

If you're dealing with recurrent cancer, you must refocus your mind from "getting a cure" for the disease to ways of "living with it." Physicians may make the analogy that ovarian cancer is like diabetes. Although both can be fatal if not treated appropriately, neither should be considered a death sentence, and the potential for living productive lives despite these diagnoses really does exist.

If you're dealing with recurrent cancer, you must refocus your mind from "getting a cure" for the disease to ways of "living with it."

Fortunately, a number of drugs are available to treat ovarian cancer. In fact, physicians can even use some drugs (the taxanes, particularly) at different doses and schedules successfully. With appropriate use of these drugs, allowing for **treatment holidays** when the cancer appears to be under control, patients can expect to live for years.

Treatment holiday

A break in treatment that allows the body time to recover from toxicity.

76. Do anti-hormone therapies have a role in treating the cancer?

Epithelial ovarian cancer is not considered to be estrogen-driven. It's true that estrogen receptors are found on this cancer, but their role in disease spread or recurrence is not clear. In addition, we know now that the use of estrogen replacement therapy doesn't negatively influence your survival. Surprisingly, though, we also know that hormone blockade can be helpful in the chronic management of ovarian cancer. Such drugs as tamoxifen, which blocks the effects of estrogen on cells, have been used in ovarian cancer patients and in women with advanced disease. Up to 15% of women given tamoxifen will have a response. Oncologists have also used other hormone blockade drugs in the treatment of chronic ovarian cancer (see **Table 5,** Question 73).

Nonepithelial ovarian cancers (e.g., granulosa-cell tumors) also can be hormonally driven, and physicians should avoid the use of estrogen. In fact, the drug **leuprolide acetate** (see **Table 5,** Question 73) has been shown to be active in the treatment of granulosa-cell tumors.

Leuprolide acetate

An anti-hormone that blocks release of estrogen and progesterone at the level of the brain.

77. What treatments are available if my cancer comes back?

Multiple options are available for treating recurrent ovarian cancer; the choice depends largely on your treatment-free interval (TFI). For platinum-based agents the outcome from re-treatment is influenced by the TFI, and the response rate can range from 27% if the TFI is 1 year to 77% if the TFI is longer than 2 years.

If you have a TFI of 3 to 6 months, the chance of a response to carboplatin is not that high. In such situations, most oncologists would recommend using a drug that works differently than carboplatin.

Fortunately, many drugs that are active in treating ovarian cancer can be tried. These include liposomal doxorubicin (Doxil), topotecan (Hycamtin), gemcitabine (Gemzar), docetaxel (Taxotere), vinorelbine (Navelbine); hexamethylamine (Hexalen); and etoposide (VePesid; see **Table 6**). In addition, clinical trials (tests involving patients and experimental drugs) continue to explore new ways of fighting ovarian cancer, and such trials are open to patients throughout the country in cancer centers and major research institutions.

It is important at this point to clarify how drugs are prescribed. There are three types of drugs that might be used to treat ovarian cancer. The first kind is the experimental drugs which have not been approved for use by the Food and Drug Administration (FDA) and cannot be prescribed outside of a clinical trial, unless a physician gets a "compassionate use" waiver for a patient who has run out of options. The second kind includes all drugs that have completed clinical trials in ovarian cancer patients and were found to be effective; these drugs have been given the stamp of approval for use in ovarian cancer patients, although the approval is sometimes qualified—that is, they may be approved for use in one stage of the disease but possibly not for another. The third kind is a gray area: drugs that have been approved for use in a similar disease (for example, breast cancer) but not for ovarian cancer. Such drugs may be prescribed "off-label"—that is, not in accordance with the rather stringent FDA indications—if the physician has reason to believe they might be effective. This is not as much of a stretch as it might sound. In many cases, very similar drugs are approved for use in ovarian cancer, but the particular drug being prescribed off-label simply hasn't gotten through sufficient trials to ascertain the proper dose, its effectiveness for a given stage of cancer, or that it is more effective and/or less toxic than the standard approved drugs. Looking at Table 6, you'll see, for example, that the drug paclitaxel is approved for ovarian cancer, although docetaxel is not. Both are taxanes, and both are effective against similar cancers, so it's entirely possible that docetaxel could work against ovarian cancer—but it's not approved. Only by going through (and passing) the rigorous testing required by the FDA will it gain that approval.

It's important to keep in mind that although the goal of treatment for recurrent cancer is to induce a remission of the cancer, the chance of a permanent remission (cure) for

Table 6 Standard drugs used in chemotherapy for ovarian cancer

Agent	Activity	Route of Infusion	Major Side Effects
Platinum analogs	Cross-link DNA, lead ulti-mately to DNA damage and cell death		
Cisplatin[A]		By vein every 3 weeks	Nausea, vomiting; numbness, tingling that may not be reversible; kidney injury; hearing loss; ringing in the ears (tinnitus)
Carboplatin[A]		By vein every 3 weeks	Lowered platelet count and white blood cell count; possible infection; nausea (less than with cisplatin); mild numbness, tingling; low risk for hearing problems
Taxanes	Inhibits cells from dividing by binding microtubules		
Paclitaxel[A]		By vein either as 1-hour infusion weekly; 3-hour infusion (if given with carboplatin) every 3 weeks; or 24-hour infusion every 3 weeks (if given with cisplatin)	Allergic reactions; complete hair loss; muscle and joint pain; numbness, tingling (reversed when drug is stopped); lowers white cell count
Docetaxel[O]		By vein as 1-hour infusion, every week or every three weeks.	Allergic reactions; lowered white cell count; hair loss; diarrhea; fluid retention

(continued)

Table 6 Standard drugs used in chemotherapy for ovarian cancer (continued)

Agent	Activity	Route of Infusion	Major Side Effects
Vinca alkaloids	Stop cells from multiplying by binding cell structures called tubulin		
Vincristine,[O] vinblastine,[O] vinorelbine[O]		By vein every 2–3 weeks (vincristine, vinblastine); every 1–2 weeks (vinorelbine)	Skin and soft-tissue damage from leaks into skin; numbness, tingling; constipation (severe with vinblastine); nausea; hair loss; lowered white blood cells
Topoisomerase inhibitors	Stabilize DNA with enzyme (topoisomerase), leads to DNA damage and cell death		
Topotecan[A]		By vein weekly or daily for 5 days every 3 weeks	Lowered red and white blood cells, platelets; hair loss, fatigue, or rash (less common)
Irinotecan[O]		By vein, usually weekly for 4 weeks, then 2 weeks off (i.e., 6-week cycle)	Significant diarrhea; lowered white blood cells or platelets hair loss nausea, vomiting lung injury
Etoposide[O]		Orally for 3 of 4 weeks	Lowered white blood cells and platelets; nausea, vomiting; hair loss; leukemia reported in women previously treated with etoposide

(continued)

Table 6 Standard drugs used in chemotherapy for ovarian cancer (continued)

Agent	Activity	Route of Infusion	Major Side Effects
Anthracycline antibiotics	Interrupts DNA, leads to cell death		
Doxorubicin[A]		By vein every 3 weeks	Serious tissue injury from intravenous line leak; lowered white blood cells, platelets; heart failure
Liposomal doxorubicin[A]		By vein every 4 weeks	Painful rash on palms and soles; acute infusion reaction (flushing, chills, back pain, shortness of breath, lowered blood pressure), generally resolves with interruption of infusion
Antimetabolites	Incorporates into DNA and leads to DNA damage and cell death		
Capecitabine[O]		Orally twice daily for 2 of 3 weeks	Lowered red and white blood cells, platelets; nausea or vomiting; diarrhea or constipation; abdominal pain; rash on hands and feet
Gemcitabine[O]		By vein weekly for 3 of 4 weeks	Lowered white blood cells, platelets; rash; shortness of breath; flu-like syndrome; mild nausea

(continued)

Relapse

Table 6 Standard drugs used in chemotherapy for ovarian cancer (continued)

Agent	Activity	Route of Infusion	Major Side Effects
Antitumor antibiotics			
Bleomycin[O]	Breaks DNA in presence of copper, iron, and cobalt; causes cell death	By vein weekly	Lung toxicity (possibly fatal); fever; oral ulcers; hair loss; skin darkening; anorexia; lowered blood cell counts
Alkylating agents	Disrupt DNA, cause cell death		
Altretamine[A]		Orally four times daily for 14–21 days	Nausea, vomiting; numbness, tingling; lowered blood cell counts
Melphalan[A]		Orally for 4 days every 4–6 weeks	Lowered blood cell counts; possible leukemia later in life
Chlorambucil[O]		Orally for 5–14 days	Lowered blood cell counts; nausea, vomiting; leukemia risk later in life
Cyclophosphamide[A]		By vein every 3 weeks	Nausea, vomiting; lowered blood cell counts; bladder bleeding (hemorrhagic cystitis); hair loss

[A]FDA approved for use in ovarian cancer.

[O]Approved for other uses but sometimes prescribed off-label for ovarian cancer.

recurrent ovarian cancer does not exist—yet. Do not forget that advances in cancer treatment are occurring continually, so that a new, more effective treatment for recurrent ovarian cancer could be just around the corner. Currently, the aim of treating recurrent ovarian cancer is to prevent or minimize cancer-related symptoms by decreasing the amount of tumor present. The major challenge in choosing a treatment is to choose an active drug that will not cause more symptoms than those caused by the cancer itself.

78. Is there any way to choose which chemotherapy option will work best for me?

There are several tests currently available or in development to predict either chemotherapy resistance (which drugs are unlikely to work for you) or chemotherapy sensitivity (which drugs are more likely to be effective for you). In general they require fresh samples (usually tumor biopsies or fluid samples from ascites or pleural effusions), which are then exposed to different drugs (and combinations of drugs) in a laboratory setting in order to see with which drugs your cancer grows despite being exposed to them (testing for resistance) or which drugs can kill it best (sensitivity). If you are predicted to be resistant to certain drugs, then your physician may avoid them because they are not likely to work.

Despite the promise of these tumor resistance assays, their role in the management of ovarian cancer remains unclear. A recent statement by the American Society of Clinical Oncology reviewed the evidence for the use of these assays and concluded that there was not sufficient evidence that they improved survival. Therefore, at this point, they are considered investigational and not recommended for routine management decisions.

79. How do you decide between using a combination of drugs or single agent chemotherapy?

Earlier, we discussed the importance of the treatment-free interval (TFI) in helping decide about re-treatment with a platinum agent. The TFI is also useful in helping to make decisions about whether to use combination or single-agent chemotherapy. In women who have platinum-resistant disease (defined as a recurrence less than 6 months after the end of the first-line treatment), the standard of care is to use single agents. Most oncologists will treat with drugs with a different mechanism of action from the platinums or the taxanes, such as pegylated liposomal doxorubicin (PLD; Doxil), topotecan, or hexamethylalamine. Combination therapy is usually discouraged in women who have early recurrence after platinum-based treatment because the likelihood that it will help improve survival is not very high.

Women with a TFI over 12 months are considered platinum-sensitive, and for this group there is a possibility of a prolonged second remission. Most oncologists agree that re-treatment with a platinum-based combination is reasonable. Data from Europe showed that in these women carboplatin and paclitaxel were better than single-agent carboplatin. Other probably useful platinum-based combinations include carboplatin and gemcitabine or carboplatin and PLD. Both of these combinations have data to suggest that they may be reasonable alternatives to carboplatin and paclitaxel.

For women who recur between 6 and 12 months, re-treatment with carboplatin can be considered as well, because it's likely that their tumor will be platinum-sensitive. Still, some oncologists may opt to treat with a nonplatinum drug and "prolong" the platinum-free interval. That way, it is hoped that the next time platinum is used there will be a better chance of a response. Artificially prolonging the TFI has not been examined well in clinical trials.

Women with a TFI of less than 6 months are considered platinum-resistant. For these women, combination therapy is generally not recommended because there is very little chance that combination therapy will induce a remission. In these women, the goals of treatment are to obtain a response, or at least disease stability, while preserving quality of life. Therefore, single-agent treatment is recommended. As long as your cancer isn't growing on treatment and the side effects are tolerable, it is usually continued.

80. Are there risks with re-treatment using carboplatin?

It is recognized that between 5% and 34% of women undergoing re-treatment with carboplatin the second time around will experience an allergic reaction to carboplatin. Curiously, it often occurs during the second re-treatment cycle (or eighth cumulative cycle). The symptoms of an allergic reaction can range from mild (redness or itching) to severe (changes in blood pressure and difficulty breathing) to full-blown anaphylaxis. There is no way to predict who is going to have an allergic reaction to carboplatin, so monitoring during re-treatment is critical. If you do experience an allergic reaction to carboplatin, it does not necessarily mean you can never receive it again. However, the risks and the potential benefits of further platinum treatment should be re-evaluated to see if further treatment makes sense.

There are case reports of death during treatment with a platinum after an allergic reaction developed. Because of this, recent studies have evaluated the use of desensitization protocols with carboplatin. Desensitization describes the process of a slow and gradual re-exposure to the drug with the intent of not triggering an allergic reaction. It has been used historically as a way to re-treat penicillin-allergic patients. The same approach has been used successfully with carboplatin, and this approach is recommended if the decision is made to continue platinum therapy. However, if your reaction is very serious (anaphylaxis, for example) then carboplatin rechallenge may not be recommended.

81. If my cancer goes into remission, what can I do to increase my chances that it won't come back again?

Recent data suggest that a second remission only rarely will be as long as the first. In addition, there are no standard treatments to maintain a remission. This has prompted many different research programs throughout the country to find ways of extending the time of remission. These programs may use chemotherapy or more novel treatments, such as immunotherapy or vaccines, to maintain remission. If you are interested in being as aggressive as possible to prevent or delay a recurrence, we would encourage you to research these options available on a clinical trial.

82. How long will I live now that my cancer has recurred?

This question is the one nearly every patient with cancer asks (or worries about, even if she doesn't ask it), but it's almost impossible to predict how much time a specific patient will have. The fact is that some women will die quickly from their cancer, whereas others will live well beyond 5 years, and there's no predicting who will live longer and who won't. Some patients given prognoses of a few months live for years longer than their doctors expected. Most clinical trials show that survival from a diagnosis of recurrence ranges from 40% to 84% at 3 years. However, we must emphasize that many factors must be taken into consideration for each individual patient. You shouldn't try to apply these statistics to your specific cancer and situation. Remember, too, that your doctor's prognosis of "2 to 3 years" is made without any knowledge of future scientific breakthroughs. There are plenty of people alive today whose doctors predicted short lifespans for them initially—people whose lives were saved by the creation of

It's almost impossible to predict how much time a specific patient will have.

new forms of cancer therapy that work well on even advanced cancers. So take any predictions about your future with a big grain of salt, because medicine, like everything else, changes very rapidly.

Dealing with recurrent cancer is about more than simply living as long as possible, however. An important aspect of the prognosis is knowing how much good time you have left to you, also referred to as "quality of life." We can improve and lengthen your "good-quality life" by offering chemotherapy to control your cancer from spreading and to limit cancer-related symptoms; by making sure that any pain you have is addressed fully; by using every means necessary to ensure that your bowels continue to function; and by knowing when further therapy is likely to hurt you more than help you. All this must be done in the setting of an open and honest relationship with your physician.

PART SEVEN

If Treatment Fails

How do I know when it's time to stop treatment?

What is a PEG tube? Do I need one?

Does intravenous feeding play a role?

More...

83. How do I know when it's time to stop treatment?

The relationship between you and your oncologist is very important and must be built on honesty and trust. This becomes more and more important if you're dealing with recurrent ovarian cancer, particularly as different treatments become necessary to try to control your cancer. Because this is a cancer that can be controlled in many women, most patients will undergo several regimens of chemotherapy with the hope of sending the cancer into remission or at least stopping it from actively growing. In fact, it's not uncommon for patients to receive three or even more different types of chemotherapy during the course of their cancer.

One of the hardest questions to ask—and even harder to answer—is when to stop trying.

One of the hardest questions to ask—and even harder to answer—is when to stop trying. Sometimes, a patient will become too sick for further treatment, in which case the oncologist would recommend stopping. Other times, it's the patient who refuses further treatment and instead chooses to live out the rest of her life naturally.

For the majority of patients, the time to stop may be on realizing that, after multiple rounds with different types of chemotherapy, the cancer has only continued to grow and no promising agents are being used in a clinical trial (a test involving patients and drugs). However, ultimately you and your physician must make the decision to stop. If patients in this type of situation still maintain an independent lifestyle, continuing other types of novel treatment or chemotherapy may be reasonable.

Bowel obstruction

Condition where the small or large bowel is blocked due to either adhesions or tumor that causes the bowel to back up instead of work normally (to get rid of stool).

If a patient's bowels stop working, particularly if this happens after or during one of these drug regimens (programs or schedules), doctors should discontinue treatment. The reason is that chemotherapy cannot relieve a **bowel obstruction**, but it certainly can add to its complications.

84. What is a PEG tube? Do I need one?

A PEG tube is a **percutaneous endoscopic gastrostomy** tube. The name describes how and where it's placed. A stomach specialist or **gastroenterologist** would place it during a short procedure. Usually, your doctor would give you medication to make the insertion more comfortable, but it does not require that you be put to sleep, as with regular surgery.

During the procedure, the gastroenterologist will use a special fiber-optic camera, called an **endoscopic camera**, introduced through your mouth and into your stomach. Once it's in place, the specialist would pump air into your stomach so that when a light shines in the internal stomach, it can be seen outside, through the skin overlying it. The specialist would make a hole through the skin and into your stomach and, through this hole, would place a tube by passing it over the camera. It remains in place in your stomach and exits through the hole in your skin.

The main purpose of a PEG tube is to provide continuous stomach drainage in patients who have a bowel obstruction due to cancer growing around the small intestines and in whom surgery cannot be performed for technical reasons. A PEG tube is not placed in everyone who has ovarian cancer. It's usually reserved for patients whose cancer is very advanced and who suffer from continual vomiting caused by gastric juices backing up from the bowels because of an intestinal obstruction (blockage). The PEG tube allows the fluid to exit the body more easily, which helps the patient to stop vomiting.

The PEG tube is usually permanent and is attached to a drainage bag into which the stomach contents are drained continuously. Women who have PEG tubes can continue to drink liquids, but whatever is not absorbed into their bowel exits through the PEG tube, instead of coming back up as

Percutaneous endoscopic gastrostomy (PEG)

A tube placed by a gastroenterologist that is inserted through your skin (percutaneous) and into your stomach.

Gastroenterologist

A medical specialist in treating disorders of the esophagus, stomach, bowel, and rectum.

Endoscopic camera

A flexible camera within a tube (the endoscope) that is used to do minimally invasive procedures.

vomit. Women with PEG tubes can also enjoy independence, because the bag to which the PEG tube is attached can be attached to the patient's leg.

The PEG tube is not a treatment for cancer; it's a way to relieve vomiting due to malignant intestinal obstruction, so that you're not throwing up all the time. Sometimes, if you're feeling better, your doctor might disconnect the tube so that you can take pills and eat and drink. However, if you were suddenly to feel nauseous, the tube can be allowed to drain so that you're not throwing up.

It's important to realize that not all patients require a PEG tube. It's offered only as a way to live with the cancer when it's far advanced and the treatments are no longer keeping it under control. As a consequence, it's used only in the most advanced cases when the disease is considered terminal.

85. Does intravenous feeding play a role?

Total parenteral nutrition (TPN)

Nutrition that is given by vein.

Intravenous feeding, or **total parenteral nutrition (TPN)**, is usually reserved for women when they first get sick with their cancer. Surgeons use TPN to help to provide nourishment to their patient to make the aggressive up-front treatments of surgery and chemotherapy more manageable.

However, the role of TPN for women with recurrent ovarian cancer is more controversial. If the cancer is growing to the point at which the patient can no longer eat or drink, TPN is probably of very little value. A recent study from Women & Infants' Hospital in Providence suggested that women with advanced ovarian cancer who were on TPN had a shorter overall survival time than women not receiving TPN.

Its use requires an indwelling (permanently placed) intravenous line or MediPort and can cause complications (e.g., clotting) due to the catheter, metabolic problems, and infections. More importantly, it has not been found to improve the life span of advanced cancer patients, nor has it been shown to offer much in the way of relieving hunger or thirst. In one study of patients with different types of cancer receiving TPN, patients with ovarian cancer given home TPN had the shortest survival rate, compared to similar patients with colon cancer or appendiceal primaries.

In individual situations, TPN may be offered, but that option must take place only after a thoughtful discussion among you, your family, and your doctor. Such a frank discussion should take into account the pros and cons of TPN in the context of how you're doing at the time.

86. What is hospice?

Hospice is also known as **palliative** care or end-of-life care. When treatments are no longer working and a patient becomes very sick because of her cancer, the doctor may recommend hospice. It represents a concerted effort by doctors and other health care providers to recognize that the end of life is a part of the disease process. We have a responsibility to help the patient and her family to remain as comfortable as possible with dignity and free of pain. Hospice care can be delivered either in an inpatient facility (either a hospital or nursing home–type setting) or at home.

Palliation

To provide relief of pain. Adj.: palliative.

Often, providers make an attempt to honor the wishes of a patient. If a woman chooses to go home to live out the rest of her life, providers can set up hospice services to meet her needs and address issues of pain and comfort. They also try to take into account the concerns of her family. However, if the patient's needs are too much for the family to handle or if she's too sick to go home, her health care providers may recommend inpatient hospice. The ultimate goal is to provide a peaceful death when a patient reaches the end stages of cancer.

87. What is a DNR order?

DNR stands for "do not resuscitate." This order represents your wishes in case something happens to you that, without the use of machines, you would likely die. If you were unable to speak for yourself, this order will help your family, your physician, or your health care proxy to make decisions for you when that time comes. In this order, you would be asked to state specifically what you would want done and what you would not want done if you were to have a life-threatening event.

These decisions are in large part state-determined. For example, in Connecticut, a DNR order must specify clearly if you do or do not want to have a tube inserted into your throat to help you breathe (**intubation**), cardiac resuscitation, intravenous fluids, or total parenteral nutrition (TPN). In New York, both intubation and cardiac resuscitation are included in the DNR order.

Intubation

Process by which a person is placed on a breathing machine.

You should not wait to establish a DNR order until you become so sick that you have to make the decision without having time to really think about it or you are considered terminal. The best time to discuss it is when you are still healthy, so that you and your family can ask questions and thoroughly talk it over with your doctor.

It's important to realize that a DNR order is not permanent. If at any point you change your mind regarding what you would want for yourself in a life-threatening situation, your health care team and your family must respect your wishes.

88. What is a health care proxy?

A health care proxy is a person whom you designate to make health care decisions for you in the event that you are unable to tell your physicians your wishes. This can be a very important role, so it's important for you as a patient to initiate a discussion of what you would want for yourself. Only then can your physicians make sure that they're abiding by your wishes. If you don't designate a health care proxy, your family often has to make decisions for you. Doing that can be risky because, although they may be acting with your best interests at heart, their decisions may not necessarily be what you would want. In addition, it's not uncommon for different members of your family to disagree with each other, particularly when it comes to someone they love. By designating a health care proxy, your family and loved ones would know that you specifically chose someone to speak for you.

89. What are the end stages of ovarian cancer like?

Ovarian cancer usually causes problems by spreading through-out the abdomen and pelvis. Although cancer can involve the brain, lungs, and liver, most women die of disease affecting their bowels. Obstruction of the large bowel (the colon) can lead to problems with bowel movements, causing constipa-tion. This can cause the colon to become very large, much like a balloon, also called **colonic dilation**. If it persists, it can become an emergency and result in a tear in the bowel, called a **perforation**. In that event, a surgeon may recommend emergency surgery to deal with the obstruction.

The cancer can also obstruct the small bowel and result in problems when the patient tries to eat. This results in nausea and vomiting of food; if not eating, a patient may also vomit up bile. This, too, can be very painful and may require a **naso-gastric (NG) tube** initially and a PEG tube (discussed in detail in Question 84) if it does not resolve.

Tumor growth in the belly can also block the flow of urine. When the urine backs up into the kidneys, the kidneys and the tubes that attach the kidneys to the bladder (the **ureters**) can become enlarged, called **hydronephrosis** if only the kid-neys are enlarged or **hydroureteronephrosis** if the ureter is also involved. Although this condition can cause some pain, it

Colonic dilation

Swelling of the bowel due to gas or liquid that cannot move through.

Perforation

Rupture of the wall of the bowel.

Nasogastric (NG) tube

A tube placed temporarily through the nose (naso) into the stomach (gastric) to help relieve continuous vomiting caused by a bowel obstruction.

Ureter

The anatomical struc-ture that enables us to get rid of urine. It connects the kidney to the bladder.

Hydronephrosis

Abnormal enlarge-ment of the kidney.

Hydrouretero-nephrosis

Abnormal enlargement of the kidney and the tube where urine flows, called the ureter.

Fistulas

Abnormally formed channels between two otherwise separate organs, such as between the vagina and bladder (vesicovaginal) or between the bowel and the skin (enterocutaneous).

may not cause any symptoms at all. However, it can cause the kidneys to stop working if it goes on for a long time. Other problems can include the development of channels between the bowel and the skin or bladder, called **fistulas**.

PART EIGHT

Prevention, Screening, and Advocacy

Can I protect myself from getting ovarian cancer?

Can I get ovarian cancer if I've had my ovaries removed?

Will fertility drugs increase my risk of ovarian cancer?

More...

PREVENTION

90. Can I protect myself from getting ovarian cancer?

The only way to prevent developing ovarian cancer is to have your ovaries removed. However, for women who want to have children or at least want the ability to have children in the future, that's not an option. Also, because this is a relatively uncommon disease, there's a strong possibility that a lot of women who would never have gotten ovarian cancer would go through the procedure unnecessarily. Right now, having your ovaries removed to prevent ovarian cancer (termed a **prophylactic oophorectomy**) is reserved for women considered to be at high risk for developing ovarian cancer. Oral contraceptives, or birth control pills, also can provide protection against the development of ovarian cancer.

Prophylactic oophorectomy

Removal of a woman's ovaries in an attempt to reduce or remove a risk for ovarian cancer in the future.

91. Can I get ovarian cancer if I've had my ovaries removed?

Technically speaking, having your ovaries removed will prevent you from getting ovarian cancer. However, removing your ovaries cannot prevent **primary peritoneal cancer**, which behaves similarly and is treated in the same way. It turns out that the cells that line the peritoneum are the same cells that line the ovaries. Thus, cancer can arise out of the peritoneal lining. Although this cancer is much rarer than ovarian cancer, having your ovaries removed can't prevent it.

Primary peritoneal cancer

Cancer that arises from the lining of the gut, or the peritoneum. This cancer behaves similarly to ovarian cancer and is treated much in the same way.

This happened to my cousin. She had a hysterectomy for endometriosis and was diagnosed with peritoneal cancer two years later. We now know that she's BRCA-1+, but at the time no one suspected. So BRCA-1+ women who have prophylactic surgery should be forewarned that although it reduces their risks of getting ovarian cancer, it's not a guarantee. —Marsha Posusney

92. Will fertility drugs increase my risk of getting ovarian cancer?

Although taking fertility medications is suspected of increasing one's risk of ovarian cancer by causing your ovaries to make more eggs, no conclusive evidence suggests that this is true. Certainly, there is a concern that hyperstimulation of the ovary can predispose to the development of ovarian cancer, owing to the frequent shedding of the ovarian surface, but this has yet to be proven.

SCREENING

93. Can ovarian cancer be inherited?

Yes, ovarian cancer can be inherited, but it's important to know that the majority of cases of ovarian cancer are not inherited. In fact, estimates figure that only 10% of all ovarian cancers are hereditary.

Generally, a hereditary cancer syndrome is suspected if, at the age of diagnosis, a patient is younger than age 40; has a history of prior breast cancer; or has a strong family history of other cancers, particularly in the immediate family. This having been said, certain well-recognized cancer syndromes run in families and are associated with an increased risk of ovarian cancer.

The most common hereditary cancer syndrome is the hereditary breast-ovarian cancer (HBOC) syndrome. If three or more cases of cancer are found within your immediate family (**first-degree relatives**) along with a history of four or more early-age breast cancer cases or a history of ovarian cancer at any age, clinically your family has an HBOC syndrome. Most of the cases of this syndrome are due to mutations in one of two genes, called BRCA-1 and BRCA-2. The BRCA-1 gene has been found on chromosome 17; BRCA-2 is located on chromosome 13. The mutations within these genes may confer

First-degree relatives

Blood relatives of your immediate family (father, mother, sister, or brother).

a risk for different types of cancers, but both are specifically associated with an increase in breast and ovarian cancer.

In addition to breast and ovarian cancer, these mutations are associated with an increased risk of other cancers. BRCA-1 mutation carriers may have an increased risk of colon cancer and prostate cancer (in men). BRCA-2 mutation carriers have an increased risk of male breast cancer, prostate cancer, malignant melanoma, and cancers of the pancreas, colon, gallbladder, and stomach.

Another syndrome found to exist in certain families is termed the Lynch II syndrome, which is a subtype of hereditary nonpolyposis colon cancer (HNPCC) syndrome. Such families contain multiple family members with colon cancer and cancers of the uterus. However, in addition to harboring these two, they are known to have members who have had breast cancer, ovarian cancer, and other types of cancer. These include cancers of the brain, stomach, and small bowel; leukemias; and sarcomas. The HNPCC syndrome is associated with mutations in human mismatch repair genes that are responsible for correcting errors or mutations in our DNA.

The final type of cancer syndrome associated with ovarian cancer is termed a site-specific ovarian cancer syndrome. This syndrome is seen in families with multiple members who develop only ovarian cancer. Researchers have not completely worked out the genetic explanation for this syndrome, although a proportion of these tumors may end up being due to BRCA-related mutations. Although these families' members have only ovarian cancer, their female members are still considered at risk for breast cancer. Recent data suggest that the opposite may not be true—women with a strong family history of breast cancer but not ovarian cancer were followed in a recently published study from Memorial Sloan-Kettering Cancer Center and were not found to have an increased incidence of ovarian cancer.

94. Should I have genetic counseling? How do you determine who should go for genetic testing?

If you have a family history of ovarian or breast cancer (or both) you're at increased risk of ovarian cancer. For you, genetic counseling makes sense, especially if you have sisters or young children and you're worried that they may have inherited a gene mutation. In addition, if you have a strong family history of multiple types of cancers, getting genetic counseling may make sense.

If you have a family history of ovarian or breast cancer (or both) you're at increased risk of ovarian cancer.

If you have two first-degree (immediate family) relatives (i.e., mother and sister) affected with ovarian or breast cancer, your probability of having a genetic mutation increases dramatically. The same is true if you or a first-degree relative have had both breast and ovarian cancer. A family history of colon cancer or colon polyps and ovarian cancer also raises your possibility of having a gene mutation. Finally, if your extended family history includes multiple affected members with varying types of cancer, including ovarian cancer, you may want to obtain genetic testing. If you are still unsure, it's always worthwhile to discuss genetic counseling with your doctor.

Unfortunately, being told that you have a genetic mutation associated with a cancer risk is often a double-edged sword. It may raise issues within yourself or your family as to what can be done about this risk. Should you have your breasts removed to prevent breast cancer? If you don't have ovarian cancer, should you have your ovaries removed? These surgeries when done to prevent cancer are termed prophylactic procedures. Working through such issues is difficult and makes a genetic counselor all the more important so that you can fully understand the risk of cancer in your specific situation and the potential pros and cons of prophylactic surgery.

Notably, recently published reports suggest that prophylactically removing the ovaries in women who have BRCA mutations may decrease the risk of future breast or ovarian cancer.

I know there are women who fear testing, but I think that anyone who is advised by their doctors to get it should do so. If you test positive, it can help you by qualifying you for special research and monitoring programs, and it can help your relatives, who will know to get tested if you test positive. At the moments when I'm feeling particularly down and pessimistic, it helps to think that even if I don't survive my cancer, my getting tested has probably saved the lives of the next generation in my family. —Marsha Posusney

95. Is there any way to screen for ovarian cancer?

The quick answer to this question is that there are no worthwhile screening tests for ovarian cancer for the general population. The worth of a screening program depends on three factors: the sensitivity of the test, which is the probability that a test result will be positive in a person with the disease, called the **true positive rate**; the specificity of the test, or the probability of a negative test result in a patient without the disease, called the **true negative rate**; and the prevalence of the disease, or the number of cases seen in a year. These three factors will determine the predictive value of the test.

True positive rate

The proportion of patients who have a positive test result and who do have the disease.

True negative rate

The proportion of patients who have a negative test result and who do not have the disease.

Some physicians use annual CA-125 tests and transvaginal ultrasound to look for signs of cancer in women known to be at risk. However, neither of these tests is based on good evidence, only on expert opinion. Although its accuracy has been established, the sensitivity of transvaginal ultrasound has to be taken in the context of the incidence of ovarian cancer, which is low in the general population. Thus, the predictive value of a positive ultrasound is less than 10% and increases to only 27% if combined with an elevated CA-125 result. Furthermore, screening for ovarian cancer has not been shown to result in a decrease in the mortality rate from the disease, and there remains a high risk of false-positive results.

Thus, researchers have not recommended screening in the general population. Current research is focusing on the value of screening in a group of women considered to be at high risk for ovarian cancer and on other mechanisms of early detection, including the use of novel serum markers or the use of **proteomics**. All that being said, for a woman at high risk, serial CA-125 and ultrasound every 6 months are commonly performed, but the benefit of this strategy still remains to be seen.

Proteomics

The study of protein profiles.

96. What kind of research is being conducted to cure this cancer?

The research being conducted in this field is extensive. Major efforts are under way to improve the early detection of this cancer so that we may pick it up when it hasn't spread and hence it can more likely be cured. Some of this work is exploring novel markers that may one day replace the CA-125 test as a more reliable and earlier indicator of ovarian cancer. Others are exploring the newer technologies of gene profiling (**genomics**) and protein profiling (proteomics) that may tip off doctors to the presence of cancer, even before it can show up on imaging tests.

Genomics

The study of gene expression patterns.

Work is also being done to improve surgery for ovarian cancer. Gynecological oncologists are leaders in laparoscopic surgery which may one day be an option for surgical staging (discussed in Question 17). Others are looking into more aggressive surgical operations that could obtain a higher number of women whose tumors can be optimally resected.

In addition, we continue to look for better ways to monitor our patients. The work on better imaging techniques, such as the role of PET scans, will help us in that process, particularly when the CA-125 test is not a marker of some patients' cancer. Also, the search for more effective cancer therapies continues. One day, we hope to be able to use a pill that will specifically target the cancer and not the surrounding tissue; our hope is to make the delivery (administration) of chemotherapy more convenient and, more importantly, to reduce its side effects and toxicity. Further, work continues on defining other approaches to fighting cancer, such as drugs that target new blood vessels that may feed a tumor (so-called **antiangiogenesis** agents), drugs that target the proteins that may cause the cancer to resist treatment, and newer drugs that may one day enable us to cure ovarian cancer.

Finally, researchers continue to explore ways to enable the immune system to recognize the cancer cell as foreign, so that it can kill cancer by itself. Investigators recently showed that the presence of immune cells (**T-cells**) in the cancer points to a better prognosis for patients than that obtained from tumors without T-cells. This finding supports the hypothesis that the immune system plays a role in trying to defeat or contain cancer and points to another mode of treatment that can be explored.

97. Should I research and learn more about the disease and its treatment?

When you are diagnosed with ovarian cancer, you may find yourself becoming an advocate by default—your own advocate! Indeed, it is our hope that you are reading this book because you want to know how to be proactive in your own care. When it comes to ovarian cancer, it is useful to know what you are faced with, and that is part of why this book was written. But it also helps for you to be aggressive about gathering information and asking questions. So our immediate answer to this question would be, yes, you should learn more, but do so at your own pace. Don't feel you need to become an expert overnight. Remember, too, that your emotions about your diagnosis should not be shunted aside as you pursue your ovarian cancer education. Take it slowly enough that you can absorb the information and grow comfortable with it before you continue.

Antiangiogenesis

To block new blood vessel formation.

T-cells

Immune cells that primarily fight viruses. They are being used in clinical trials of immunotherapy for ovarian and other cancers.

When it comes to ovarian cancer, it is useful to know what you are faced with.

As you grow more knowledgeable and become closely involved in your treatment, you may also find yourself becoming an advocate for others. Perhaps you will join a support group and offer support, advice, or just a badly needed ear for someone who needs to talk. Just as teachers learn their subject better through teaching, this sort of advocacy can help you as well as help others. If you want to take it a step further, consider volunteering for an advocacy organization such as those listed in the Appendix, where you can work to raise awareness of the disease or lobby for funding in support of research. If you have the energy and the inclination for this activity, it can prove helpful not only to ovarian cancer patients in general, but also to you specifically. For instance, you would be in a position to know of advances in treatment when they first become available, rather than waiting for your doctor to hear of them and recommend them to you. Again, this depends on how you as an individual feel about these activities; public advocacy is not for everyone, no matter what its advantages.

Whatever road you take, be it personal education or public advocacy, be aware of one drawback: There is so much information and so much data out there that it is not uncommon for women to get lost in the statistics. It is all too easy to forget that statistics are generalizations about ovarian cancer that, like most statistics, are so broad they are meaningless for an individual. Take them too seriously, and you may find them overwhelming. Try to find methods that will work for you without making you anxious or depressed about your disease.

98. Where can I get support?

You can consider a cancer diagnosis sort of like an invitation to join an exclusive women's club that you never expected or desired to join. This is an important concept because it relays a very important message: **You are not alone.** An entire community of women live with and fight this cancer; they are in a situation similar to yours, no matter where you are along the cancer path; and they are available to you for advice, support, or just helping with the day-to-day struggles of life with cancer. In addition, support groups are available in most local communities. We who treat cancer know that this is a disease that has an impact not only on a patient, but also on everyone who cares about her and loves her. Your nurses are often the best source of information, and they should be able to direct you toward these support groups locally or to a therapist, in case you need to talk things out in a safe and private environment. As cancer care providers, we're here not only to help you manage your cancer, but also to help you deal with the fear and questions that accompany it.

Your nurses are often the best source of information.

99. When should I ask for help?

Being diagnosed with ovarian cancer is an incredibly scary process, and no one should go through it alone. If you're feeling isolated and scared, you should reach out for support. Sadness and anxiety are common in women who have just been told that they have cancer. Most women tell me that they feel it's a death sentence and only remember what they read about Gilda Radner's brave but short struggle with this cancer. If you don't discuss them, the fears can build and make the work that must be done too hard. They can also cause a worsening sense that you're alone, and that feeds into a cycle of deepening despair. If this describes what you or someone you love is going through, reach out for help.

Such feelings must be brought out into the open. Anyone diagnosed with ovarian cancer must want to fight it and must trust that treatments are available and successful and can give you back your life. Even if the cancer comes back, there's reason to be hopeful.

Often, antidepressant and antianxiety medications are necessary to help you to come to grips with a cancer diagnosis and the change it requires in your life. Medications to help you handle the diagnosis, its challenges, and treatment are not signs of weakness. There are resources available to enable you to regain control of your life so that you can handle the decisions important to fighting this disease.

100. Where can I get more information?

Many resources are available for women newly diagnosed or living with a diagnosis of ovarian cancer. These include the organizations, Web sites, and books listed on the following pages. Many more resources are available besides those listed here; check your local library or Amazon.com for books, or go to any of the following organizations' Web sites and search for links or resources related to ovarian cancer.

Appendix

Organizations

American Academy of Medical Acupuncture
4929 Wilshire Boulevard, Suite 428
Los Angeles, CA 90010
Phone: 323-937-5514
Web site: www.medicalacupuncture.org

American Cancer Society
1599 Clifton Road
Atlanta, GA 30329
Phone: 800-ACS-2345
Web site: www.cancer.org

American Society of Clinical Oncology
1900 Duke Street, Suite 200
Alexandria, VA 22314
Phone: 703-299-0150
Web site: www.asco.org

Cancer Care, Inc.
275 Seventh Avenue
Floor 22
New York, NY 10001
Phone: 212-712-8400 (Admin); 212-712-8080 (Services)
Web site: www.cancercare.org
Page specific to ovarian cancer: www.cancercare.org/get_help/help_by_
diagnosis/diagnosis.php?diagnosis=ovarian

Cancer Research Institute
681 Fifth Avenue
New York, NY 10022
Phone: 800-99-CANCER (800-992-2623)
Web site: www.cancerresearch.org

Centers for Disease Control and Prevention
1600 Clifton Road
Atlanta, GA 30333
Phone: 404-639-3534
Toll-free: 800-311-3435
Web site: www.cdc.gov

Department of Veterans Affairs
Veterans Health Association
810 Vermont Avenue, N.W.
Washington, DC 20420
Phone: 202-273-5400 (Washington, DC office)
Toll-free: 800-827-1000 (Local VA office)
Web site: www.va.gov

FertileHOPE
P.O. Box 624
New York, NY 10014
Web site: www.fertilehope.org

Gilda's Club Worldwide
322 Eighth Avenue, Suite 1402
New York, NY 10001
Phone: 888-GILDA-4-U
Web site: www.gildasclub.org

Gynecologic Cancer Foundation
401 N. Michigan Avenue
Chicago, IL 60611
Phone: 312-644-6610
Fax: 312-527-6658
Web site: www.wcn.org/gcf

Health Insurance Association of America
555 13th Street, N.W., Suite 600
East Washington, DC 20004-1109
Web site: www.hiaa.org
Phone: 202-824-1600

Health Resources and Services Administration—Hill-Burton Program
U.S. Department of Health and Human Services
Parklawn Building

5600 Fishers Lane

Rockville, MD 20857

Phone: 301-443-5656

Toll-free: 800-638-0742/800-492-0359 (From the Maryland area)

Web site: www.hrsa.gov/osp/dfcr/about/aboutdiv.htm

Institute of Certified Financial Planners

Phone: 303-759-4900

Toll-free: 800-282-7526 (Automated referral service)

Web site: www.icfp.org

National Cancer Institute

National Cancer Institute Public Information Office

Building 31, Room 10A31

31 Center Drive, MSC 2580

Bethesda, MD 20892-2580

Phone: 301-435-3848 (Public Information Office line)

Web site: www.cancer.gov

National Cancer Institute's Cancer Trials site lists current clinical trials that have been reviewed by the NCI: http://www.cancer.gov/clinicaltrials/

National Center for Complementary and Alternative Medicine

NCCAM Clearinghouse

P.O. Box 7923

Gaithersburg, MD 20898

Phone: 888-644-6226

Web site: www.nccam.nih.gov

National Comprehensive Cancer Network

50 Huntingdon Pike, Suite 200

Rockledge, PA 19046

Phone: 888-909-NCCN (888-909-6226)

Web site: www.nccn.org

National Ovarian Cancer Coalition

500 NE Spanish River Boulevard, Suite 14

Boca Raton, FL 33431

Phone: 561-393-0005

Toll-free: 888-OVARIAN

Fax: 561-393-7275

Web site: www.ovarian.org

National Viatical Association of America
1200 19th Street, N.W.
Washington, DC 20036-2412
Phone: 202-429-5129
Toll-free: 800-741-9465
Web site: www.nationalviatical.org

National Women's Health Information Center
U.S. Department of Health and Human Services
8550 Arlington Boulevard, Suite 300
Fairfax, VA 22031
Phone: 800-994-9662
Web site: www.4women.gov

Office of Minority Health
U.S. Department of Health and Human Services
P.O. Box 37337
Washington, DC 20013-7337
Phone: 800-444-6472
Web site: www.omhrc.gov

Ovarian Cancer National Alliance
910 17th Street, N.W., Suite 1190
Washington, DC 20006
Phone: 202-331-1332
Fax: 202-331-2292
Web site: www.ovariancancer.org

SHARE
1501 Broadway, Suite 1720
New York, NY 10036
Phone: 212-719-0364 or 866-891-2392
Web site: www.sharecancersupport.org

Social Security Administration
Office of Public Inquiries
6401 Security Boulevard., Room 4-C-5 Annex
Baltimore, MD 21235-6401
Toll-free: 800-772-1213 or 800-325-0778 (TTY)
Web site: www.ssa.gov

Society of Gynecologic Oncologists
401 N. Michigan Avenue
Chicago, IL 60611
Phone: 312-644-6610
Web site: www.sgo.org

United Seniors Health Cooperative
409 3rd Street, S.W., Suite 200
Washington, DC 20024
Phone: 202-479-6973
Toll-free: 800-637-2604
Web site: www.unitedseniorshealth.org

Online Resources

CancerLinks (www.cancerlinks.org)
CancerNet (http://cancernet.nci.nih.gov)
> Detailed information provided by the National Cancer Institute on many
> types of cancer.

CancerSource (www.cancersource.com)
CancerWise/MD Anderson Cancer Center (www.cancerwise.org)
Eyes on the Prize (www.eyesontheprize.org)
> A support community for women living with gynecologic cancer.

Memorial Sloan-Kettering Cancer Center (www.mskcc.org)
SHARE (www.sharecancersupport.org)
> A support community for women and their families living with breast or
> ovarian cancer.

Women's Cancer Network (www.wcn.org)
You Are Not Alone (www.yana.org)
> Offers online and in-person support groups for those going through high-
> dose chemotherapy.

Caregivers and Home Care

Association of Cancer Online Resources
Web page: www.acor.org
Click on "Mailing Lists" and then select "Caregivers & Family Issues" for an
online discussion group for caregivers of cancer patients.

Caring for the Caregiver (National Coalition for Cancer Survivorship)
Web page: www.cansearch.org/programs/Caregiver.PDF

Family Caregiver Alliance
690 Market Street, Suite 600
San Francisco, CA 94104
Phone: 415-434-3388
Web site: www.caregiver.org
Caregiver resources include an online support group and an information clearinghouse. Information available in Spanish.

Guide for Cancer Supporters: Step-by-Step Ways to Help a Relative or Friend Fight Cancer (R.A. Bloch Cancer Foundation)
Web page: www.blochcancer.org. Click on "Info For Supporters."

National Family Caregivers Association
10400 Connecticut Avenue, #500
Kensington, MD 20895-3944
Phone: 800-896-3650
Web site: www.nfcacares.org
Provides education, information, support, and advocacy services for family caregivers.

Children

Kids Konnected
27071 Cabot Road, Suite 102
Laguna Hills, CA 92653
Phone: 949-582-5443
Web site: www.kidskonnected.org
Provides extensive support resources and programs for children who have a parent with cancer.

What Do I Tell the Children?—A Guide for a Parent with Cancer (Cancerbackup)
Web page: www.cancerbackup.org.uk/info/talk-children.htm

Clinical Trials Resources

There is no single resource for locating clinical trials for ovarian cancer. It makes sense to check all of the resources listed below repeatedly because new trials are continually added. There are also clinical trials services emerging that help to match patients to clinical trials. Some of these services can be useful for obtaining information and saving time, but it is important to read the company's privacy statement and be aware of whether the company is being paid for recruiting patients.

National Cancer Institute Clinical Trials
Phone: 800-4CANCER
Web site: www.cancer.gov/clinical_trials/
The NCI offers comprehensive information on understanding and finding
clinical trials, including access to the NCI/PDQ Clinical Trials Database.

National Institutes of Health/National Library of Medicine Clinical Trials
Web site: ClinicalTrials.gov
Clinical trials database service developed by the National Institute of Health's
National Library of Medicine.

Centerwatch Clinical Trials Listing Service
Web site: www.centerwatch.com
Listing of clinical trials conducted by drug companies.

NCI Clinical Trials and Insurance Coverage
Web page: www.cancer.gov/clinicaltrials/learning/insurance-coverage
Excellent in-depth guide to clinical trials insurance issues.

Complementary and Alternative Medicine (CAM)

American Academy of Medical Acupuncture
Web site: www.medicalacupuncture.org
Professional site with articles on acupuncture, a list of frequently asked
questions, and an acupuncturist locator.

Commonweal
P.O. Box 316
Bolinas, CA 94924
Phone: 415-868-0970
Web site: www.commonweal.org
Provides information on complementary approaches to cancer care, including
the full text of Michael Lerner's 1994 book, *Choices in Healing: Integrating the
Best of Conventional and Complementary Approaches to Cancer*, published by MIT
press (updated version available in print).

National Center for Complementary and Alternative Medicine (NCCAM)
Web site: http://nccam.nih.gov
Offers information on complementary and alternative medicine therapies,
including NCI/PDQ expert-reviewed fact sheets on individual therapies and
dietary supplements.

NCI Office of Cancer Complementary and Alternative Medicine (OCCAM)
Web site: www.cancer.gov/occam
Information clearinghouse supporting the NCI's CAM activities.

Diet and Nutrition

American Institute for Cancer Research
1759 R Street, N.W.
Washington, DC 20009
Phone: 800-843-8114 or 202-328-7744 (in DC)
Web site: www.aicr.org
Supports research on diet and nutrition in the prevention and treatment
of cancer. Provides information to cancer patients on nutrition and cancer,
including a compilation of healthy recipes. Maintains a nutrition hotline for
questions relating to nutrition and health.

Nutrition (American Cancer Society)
Web page: www.cancer.org. Enter "nutrition" in the search box.
Nutrition resources include: ACS guidelines on nutrition, dietary supplement
information, nutrition message boards, and tips on low-fat cooking and choosing
healthy ingredients.

Drugs/Medications

MedlinePlus: Drug Information
Web page: www.medlineplus.gov. Click on "Drugs & Supplements."
A guide to over 9,000 prescription and over-the-counter medications provided
by U.S. Pharmacopeia (USP).

Employment, Insurance, Financial, and Legal Resources

Organizations and Programs
Americans with Disabilities Act (U.S. Department of Justice)
Cancer Legal Resource Center
919 S. Albany Street
Los Angeles, CA 90019-10015
Phone: 213-736-1455
Web page: www.usdoj.gov/crt/ada/adahom1.htm
A joint program of Loyola Law School and the Western Law Center for
Disability Rights. Provides information and educational outreach on cancer-
related legal issues to people with cancer and others impacted by the disease.

Centers for Medicare & Medicaid Services (CMS)

(formerly the Health Care Financing Administration [HCFA])

Web site: www.cms.hhs.gov

Oversees administration of:

- Medicare—Federal health insurance program for people 65 years or older and some disabled people under 65 years of age.
  Phone: 800-633-4227
  Web site: www.medicare.gov
- Medicaid—Federal–state health insurance program for certain low-income people. Contact your state Medicaid offices for further information.
  Web page: www.cms.hhs.gov/home/medicaid.asp
- Health Insurance Portability and Accountability Act (HIPAA)—Insurance reform that may lower your chance of losing existing coverage, ease your ability to switch health plans, and/or help you buy coverage on your own if you lose your employer's plan and have no other coverage available.
  Web page: www.cms.hhs.gov/HIPAAGenInfo/

Family and Medical Leave Act (FMLA)

Web page: www.dol.gov/esa/whd/fmla/

U.S. Department of Labor web page providing information about the Family and Medical Leave Act (FMLA)

Health Insurance Association of America (HIAA)

1201 F Street, N.W., Suite 500

Washington, DC 20004-1204

Phone: 202-824-1600

Web site: www.hiaa.org/cons/cons.htm

Provides insurance guides for consumers. Topics include health insurance and managed care, disability income, long-term care, and medical savings accounts.

Hill-Burton Program (Health Resources and Services Administration)

Phone: 301-443-5656

Toll-free: 800-638-0742 (800-492-0359 in Maryland)

Web page: www.hrsa.gov/OSP/dfcr/obtain/obtain.htm

Facilities that receive Hill-Burton funds from the government are required by law to provide services to some people who cannot afford to pay. Information on Hill-Burton eligibility and facilities locations is available via phone or the Internet.

Patient Advocate Foundation
753 Thimble Shoals Boulevard, Suite B
Newport News, VA 23606
Phone: 800-532-5274
Web site: www.patientadvocate.org
Nonprofit organization helps patients to resolve insurance, debt, and job discrimination matters relative to cancer. Patient resources include *The National Financial Resources Guidebook for Patients: A State-by-State Directory*, *Your Guide to the Appeals Process*, and the *Managed Care Answer Guide*.

Social Security Administration (SSA)
Web site: www.ssa.gov
Oversees two programs that pay benefits to people with disabilities:
- Social Security Disability Insurance—Pays benefits to you and certain members of your family if you have worked long enough and paid Social Security taxes.
- Supplemental Security Income—Supplements Social Security payments based on need.

Veterans Health Administration
810 Vermont Avenue, N.W.
Washington, DC 20420
Phone: 202-273-5400 or 877-222-8387 (health care benefits)
Web site: www.va.gov/vbs/health/
Eligible veterans and their dependents may receive cancer treatment at a Veterans Administration Medical Center.

Financial Assistance Programs
Air Care Alliance
Phone: 888-260-9707
Web site: www.aircareall.org
Network of organizations willing to provide public benefit flights for health care.

Finding Ways to Pay for Care (National Coalition for Cancer Survivorship)
Web page: www.cansearch.org. Select "Programs" and then "Cancer Survival Toolbox."

NeedyMeds
Web site: www.needymeds.com
Information on patient assistance programs and other programs that help people obtain medications, supplies, and equipment.

Hospice and End-of-Life Issues

Partnership for Caring
1620 Eye Street, N.W., Suite 202
Washington, DC 20006
Phone: 202-296-8071
Toll-free: 800-989-9455
Web site: www.partnershipforcaring.org
Comprehensive information and resources covering end-of-life issues, including advance directives.

Association of Online Cancer Resources, Cancer-Hospice mailing list
Web site: www.acor.org. Click on "Mailing Lists," select "Hospice," and then select "Cancer-Hospice."
Online discussion group for cancer patients dealing with hospice issues.

Growth House
Web site: www.growthhouse.org
Extensive, annotated directory of hospice and end-of-life resources organized by topic.

Home Care Guide for Advanced Cancer (American College of Physicians)
Web page: www.acponline.org/public/h_care/
Guide for family and friends caring for advanced cancer patients who are living at home.

Hospice Net
Web site: www.hospicenet.org
Provides comprehensive information to patients and families facing life-threatening illness. Extensive resources addressing end-of-life issues from both patient and caregiver perspectives.

Patient Advocacy Skills

Cancer Survival Toolbox (National Coalition for Cancer Survivorship)
Web page: www.cansearch.org. Select "Programs" and then "Cancer Survival Toolbox."
Topics include communication skills, finding information, solving problems, making decisions, negotiating, and standing up for your rights. (Also available as audiotapes at 877-866-5748.)

Physician and Hospital Locators

American Society of Clinical Oncology (ASCO)
Web page: www.asco.org. Click on the "Find an Oncologist" button.

American College of Surgeons (ACS) Commission on Cancer
Web page: www.facs.org/cpm/default.htm
Listing of ACS Commission on Cancer's Approved Hospital Cancer Programs.

American Medical Association (AMA) DoctorFinder
Web page: www.ama-assn.org/aps/amahg.htm
Provides professional information on licensed U.S. physicians.

Prevention and Risk Assessment

Prevention (American Cancer Society)
Web page: www.cancer.org. Enter "prevention" in the search box.
Comprehensive section on prevention covers topics such as environmental and occupational cancer risks, exercise, tobacco and cancer, nutrition for risk reduction, and prevention and detection programs.

Your Cancer Risk (Harvard Center for Cancer Prevention)
Web site: www.yourdiseaserisk.harvard.edu. Click on "What's Your Cancer Risk?"
Online ovarian cancer risk assessment tool.

Research Resources and Reference

PubMed: MEDLINE (National Library of Medicine)
Web site: www.ncbi.nlm.nih.gov/PubMed/
Provides free online access to MEDLINE, a database of over 11 million citations to the medical literature.

Medscape
Web site: www.medscape.com. Enter "ovarian cancer" in the search box.
Medscape is an excellent source for the latest news in lung cancer research, including access to summaries of cancer conferences. The site is aimed at health care professionals. Registration is required for free access to Medscape.

Merriam-Webster Medical Dictionary
Web site: www.intelihealth.com. Enter "Merriam Webster" in the search box.
Registration is required for free access to Intelihealth.

Support Services

Association of Cancer Online Resources (ACOR)
Web site: www.acor.org. Click on "Mailing Lists."
ACOR offers online support groups for cancer patients.

Cancer Care
275 Seventh Avenue
New York, NY 10001
Phone: 212-712-8080
Toll-free: 800-813-4673
Web site: www.cancercare.org
Provides comprehensive support services and programs to people with cancer.

Cancer Survivors Network
Web site: www.acscsn.org
The Cancer Survivors Network is the American Cancer Society's online patient community.

R.A. Bloch Cancer Foundation
4400 Main Street
Kansas City, MO 64111
Phone: 816-932-8453
Toll-free: 800-433-0464
Web site: www.blochcancer.org
Provides Bloch-authored cancer books free of charge, a multidisciplinary referral service, and patient-to-patient phone support.

Vital Options International
15060 Ventura Boulevard, Suite 211
Sherman Oaks, CA 91403
Phone: 818-788-5225
Web site: www.vitaloptions.org
Produces "The Group Room," a weekly, syndicated radio call-in show (with simultaneous Webcast) covering important and timely topics in cancer.

Wellness Community
35 East Seventh Street, Suite 412
Cincinnati, OH 45202
Phone: 513-421-7111
Toll-free: 888-793-WELL
Web site: www.wellness-community.org
Provides educational programs and support groups for people with cancer and their families.

Talking About Cancer (American Cancer Society)
Web page: www.cancer.org. Enter "Talking About Cancer" in the search box. Discusses how to talk about your cancer with family, friends, your health care providers, and your employer. Includes resources for locating in-person and online support groups.

Coping with Cancer
Phone: 615-791-3859
Web page: www.copingmag.com
Cancer magazine available free of charge in oncology offices or by subscription.

Symptoms, Side Effects, and Complications
Fatigue
CancerFatigue.org
Web site: www.cancerfatigue.org
Information about cancer-related fatigue for patients and caregivers.

Association of Cancer Online Resources Cancer-Fatigue mailing list
Web page: www.acor.org. Click on "Mailing Lists," select "C," and then select "Cancer-Fatigue."
Online discussion list covering cancer and treatment-related fatigue.

National Comprehensive Cancer Network Cancer-Related Fatigue and Anemia Treatment Guidelines for Patients
Web page: www.nccn.org/patients/patient_gls/_english/_fatigue/contents.asp

Nausea and Vomiting
National Comprehensive Cancer Network Nausea and Vomiting Treatment Guidelines for Patients with Cancer
Web page: www.nccn.org/patient_gls/_english/_nausea_and_vomiting/contents.asp

NCI/PDQ Nausea and Vomiting
Web page: www.cancer.gov Enter "nausea" in the search box.
Expert-reviewed information summary about cancer-related nausea and vomiting.

Nutritional Problems
NCI/PDQ Nutrition
Web site: www.cancer.gov. Enter "nutrition" in the search box.
Expert-reviewed information summary about the causes and management of nutritional problems occurring in cancer patients.

Pain
The National Pain Foundation (NPF)
P.O. Box 102605
Denver, CO 80250-2605
Web site: www.NationalPainFoundation.org
The NPF Web site offers online education and support communities for pain patients and their families, including cancer pain and palliative care resources.

Association of Cancer Online Resources Cancer Pain mailing list
Web page: www.acor.org. Click on "Mailing Lists," select "C," and then select "Cancer-Pain."
Online discussion list about pain associated with cancer and its treatments.

NCCN Cancer Pain Treatment Guidelines for Patients
Web page: www.nccn.org/patients/patient_gls/_english/_pain/contents.asp

NCI/PDQ Pain
Web page: www.cancer.gov. Enter "pain" in the search box.
Expert-reviewed information summary about cancer-related pain. Includes discussion of approaches to the management and treatment of cancer-associated pain.

Peripheral Neuropathy
The Neuropathy Association
60 East 42nd Street, Suite 942
New York, NY 10165
Phone: 212-692-0662
Web site: www.neuropathy.org

Association of Cancer Online Resources Cancer-Neuropathy mailing list

Web page: www.acor.org Click on "Mailing Lists," click on "C," and then select "Cancer-Neuropathy."

Online discussion group for patients dealing with neuropathy induced by cancer or its treatments.

Almadrones, L.A., & Arcot, R. Patient Guide to Peripheral Neuropathy. *Oncology Nursing Forum.* 1999;26(8):1359–1362.

Pleural Effusion

Chemical Pleurodesis for Malignant Pleural Effusion (Cancer Supportive Care)

Web page: www.cancersupportivecare.com/pleural.html

Carolyn Clary-Macy, RN, provides a clear explanation of chemical pleurodesis for malignant pleural effusion. Aimed at patients.

Sexual Effects

Association of Cancer Online Resources Cancer-Fertility and Cancer-Sexuality mailing lists

Web site: www.acor.org. Click on "Mailing Lists," select "C," and then select "Cancer-Fertility" and/or "Cancer-Sexuality."

Online discussion lists about fertility and sexuality issues associated with cancer.

NCI/PDQ Sexuality and Reproductive Issues

Web page: www.cancer.gov. Enter "sexuality" in the search box.

Expert-reviewed information summary about factors that may affect fertility and sexual functioning in people who have cancer.

Tests and Procedures

Diagnostic Imaging (MEDLINEplus)

Web page: www.nlm.nih.gov/medlineplus/diagnosticimaging.html

Laboratory Tests (MEDLINEplus)

Web page: www.nlm.nih.gov/medlineplus/laboratorytests.html

Margolis, Simeon, ed. *The Johns Hopkins Consumer Guide to Medical Tests: What You Can Expect, How You Should Prepare, What Your Results Mean.* Baltimore, MD: The Johns Hopkins University Press, 2001.

Treatment Information and Guidelines

Chemotherapy and You (NIH/NCI)
Web page: www.cancer.gov. Enter "Chemotherapy and You" in the search box.
Also available in print by calling 800-4CANCER.

Radiation Therapy and You (NIH/NCI)
Web page: www.cancer.gov. Enter "Radiation Therapy and You" in the search
box. Also available in print by calling 800-4CANCER.

Survivorship Issues

Association of Cancer Online Resources LT-Survivors mailing list
Web page: www.acor.org. Click on "Mailing Lists," select "L," and then select
"LT-SURVIVORS."
Forum for discussion of issues of concern to long-term cancer survivors.

Books and Pamphlets

The following books are available from the American Cancer Society:
- *American Cancer Society's Guide to Complementary and Alternative Cancer Methods*
- *The American Cancer Society's Guide to Pain Control: Powerful Methods to Overcome Cancer Pain*
- *Caregiving*
- *Coming to Terms with Cancer*
- *Informed Decisions*, 2nd Edition
- *Women and Cancer*

The following pamphlets are available from the National Cancer Institute:
- *Chemotherapy and You: A Guide to Self-Help During Treatment*
- *Eating Hints for Cancer Patients Before, During, and After Treatment*
- *Get Relief from Cancer Pain*
- *Helping Yourself During Chemotherapy*
- *Questions and Answers About Pain Control: A Guide for People with Cancer and Their Families*
- *Taking Part in Clinical Trials: What Cancer Patients Need to Know*
- *Taking Time: Support for People with Cancer and the People Who Care About Them*

Available in Spanish:
- *Datos sobre el tratamiento de quimioterapia contra el cancer*
- *El tratamiento de radioterapia; guia para el paciente durante el tratamiento*
- *En que consisten los estudios clinicos? Un folleto para los pacientes de cancer*

The following pamphlets are available from the National Comprehensive Cancer Network:
- *Cancer Pain Treatment Guidelines for Patients*
- *Nausea and Vomiting Treatment Guidelines for Patient with Cancer*
- Available in Spanish: *El dolor asociado con el cáncer*

Available from The Wellness Community:
- *A Patient Active Guide to Living With Ovarian Cancer*

Books and Articles

Abrahm, JL. *A Physician's Guide to Pain and Symptom Management in Cancer Patients.* Baltimore: Johns Hopkins University Press, 2000.

American Cancer Society. *American Cancer Society's Guide to Complementary and Alternative Cancer Methods.* Atlanta, GA: American Cancer Society, 2000.

American Cancer Society. *Consumers Guide to Cancer Drugs.* Atlanta, GA: American Cancer Society, 2000.

Anderson, G. *50 Essential Things to Do When the Doctor Says It's Cancer.* New York: Penguin Books, 1993.

Benson, H. *The Relaxation Response.* New York: Avon Books, 1975.

Carney, KL. *What Is Cancer Anyway? Explaining Cancer to Children of All Ages.* Dragonfly Publishing, 1998.

Cassileth, BR. *The Alternative Medicine Handbook: The Complete Reference Guide to Alternative and Complementary Therapies.* New York: W.W. Norton & Company, 1998.

Conner, K, Langford, L, & Mayer, M. *Ovarian Cancer: Your Guide to Taking Control.* Patient-Centered Guides, 2003.

Finn, R. *Cancer Clinical Trials: Experimental Treatments & How They Can Help You.* Sebastopol, CA: O'Reilly & Associates, 1999.

Hapham, WH. *When a Parent Has Cancer: A Guide to Caring for Your Children.* New York: HarperCollins, 1997.

Harpham, WS. *After Cancer: A Guide to Your New Life.* New York: W.W. Norton & Company, 1994.

Harpham, WS. Resolving the Frustration of Fatigue. *CA: A Cancer Journal for Clinicians.* 1999;49:178–189.

Hoffman, B. *Working It Out: Your Employment Rights as a Cancer Survivor.* Silver Spring, MD: National Coalition for Cancer Survivorship, undated. This booklet can be ordered from the NCCS at 877-622-7937.

Holland, JC, & Lewis, S. *The Human Side of Cancer.* New York: HarperCollins Publishers, 2000.

Houts, PS, & Bucher, JA, eds. *Caregiving: A Step-by-Step Resource for Caring for the Person with Cancer at Home.* Atlanta, GA: American Cancer Society, 2000.

Kalter, S. 1987. *Looking Up: The Complete Guide to Looking and Feeling Good for the Recovering Cancer Patient.* Provides tips (with photos) on hair care, wigs, makeup, and exercise. (Out of print; check your local library to find a copy.)

Kaptchuk, TJ. *The Web That Has No Weaver: Understanding Chinese Medicine.* New York: McGraw-Hill, 2000.

Kohlenberg, S. 1993. *Sammy's Mommy Has Cancer.* Washington, DC: Magination Press, 1993.

Landay, DS. *Be Prepared: The Complete Financial, Legal and Practical Guide to Living with Cancer, HIV and Other Life-Challenging Conditions.* New York: St. Martin's Press, 1998.

Laughlin, EH. *Coming to Terms with Cancer: A Glossary of Cancer-Related Terms* Atlanta, GA: American Cancer Society, 2002.

McKay, J, & Hirano, N. *The Chemotherapy and Radiation Therapy Survival Guide.* Oakland, CA: New Harbinger Publications, Inc., 1998.

Mulay, M. 2002. *Making the Decision: A Cancer Patient's Guide to Clinical Trials.* Sudbury, MA: Jones & Bartlett Publishers, 2002.

Olson, K. *Surgery and Recovery*. Traverse City, MI: Rhodes & Easton, 1998.

Oster, N, et al. *Making Informed Medical Decisions: Where to Look and How to Use What You Find*. Sebastopol, CA: O'Reilly & Associates, Inc., 2000. Outstanding article by a patient/physician discusses cancer-related fatigue and how to deal with it.

Piver, MS, Wilder, G, & Bull, J. *Gilda's Disease: Sharing Personal Experiences and a Medical Perspective on Ovarian Cancer*. New York: Bantam Doubleday, 1998.

Schimmel, SR, & Fox, B. *Cancer Talk: Voices of Hope and Endurance from "The Group Room," the World's Largest Cancer Support Group*. New York: Broadway Books, 1999.

Willis, J. *The Cancer Patient's Workbook*. New York: Dorling Kindersley Publishing, Inc., 2001.

Glossary

A

Adenocarcinomas: Type of cancer, arising from the cells of epithelial origin.

Adenomas: Noncancerous tumors arising from epithelial cells.

Adhesions: Scarring within the abdominal cavity. These commonly occur in patients who have had prior surgery.

Adjuvant: Given after a primary procedure.

Anechoic: Used in ultrasound studies, describes a lack of different ultrasound signals, commonly seen with simple cysts.

Antiangiogenesis: To block new blood vessel formation.

Antigen: A protein that sits on or is released from cells that can be targeted with an antibody or a vaccine.

Antihistamine: To block the release of histamines, which are often associated with allergic reactions.

Apoptosis: Programmed cell death.

Ascites: Fluid build-up within the abdomen.

Atypia: Used by pathologists, it describes abnormal cellular changes seen under the microscope.

B

Belly wash: Common term for an intraperitoneal treatment.

Benign: Not cancerous.

Bilateral salpingo-oophorectomy: The surgical term for removal of both the right and left fallopian tubes and ovaries.

Biopsy: Removal of a small amount of tissue for analysis by a pathologist. It can be done during surgery or before surgery using other less invasive procedures.

Borderline: A term used to describe a tumor that does not appear normal but does not meet a pathologist's criteria for cancer; otherwise described as low malignant potential.

Bowel obstruction: Condition where the small or large bowel is blocked due to either adhesions or tumor that causes the bowel to back up instead of work normally (to get rid of stool).

C

Capillaries: The smallest blood vessels within your body.

Carbohydrate antigen: A type of protein released from cells.

Carcinomatosis: Cancer deposits along the abdomen, often along the bowel and involving the omentum.

Clinical complete remission: A normal physical exam, tumor marker, and radiology tests following the completion of front-line treatment for cancer.

Cognitive: Referring to the higher mental process of reasoning, thinking, remembering, and learning.

Colon: The large intestine, part of your gastrointestinal tract. Its function is to absorb water and food and to excrete stool.

Colonic dilation: Swelling of the bowel due to gas or liquid that cannot move through.

Colostomy: A loop of bowel that is pulled through your skin.

Complete resection: Removal of all the tumor in your abdomen and pelvis.

Computed tomography: Otherwise known as a CT scan, this is a highly sensitive radiology exam used to help diagnose and follow patients with cancer.

Cremaphore: A molecule to which drugs are attached to increase the drugs' delivery into your body.

Cytological analysis: The process of examining cells under the microscope; the sample is usually obtained from floating cells in the fluid of the abdomen (ascites) or chest (pleural effusions).

D

Debulking: The process of removing cancer from your body.

Differentiation: The process of cells maturing so they can perform specific processes in our bodies.

Direct extension: The process by which cancer extends into local and surrounding tissue.

Dyspnea: Shortness of breath.

E

Early satiety: Feeling of getting full faster than you normally would.

Echogenic: An ultrasound term describing complex patterns seen within a cyst.

Endodermal sinus tumor: A type of germ-cell tumor, derived from early cells destined to become eggs. Otherwise, they are referred to as yolk-sac tumors.

Endoscopic camera: A flexible camera within a tube (the endoscope) that is used to do minimally invasive procedures.

Estrogen: A female hormone produced by the ovaries; it is responsible for female changes during maturity.

F

First-degree relatives: Blood relatives of your immediate family (father, mother, sister, or brother).

Fistulas: Abnormally formed channels between two otherwise separate organs, such as between the vagina and bladder (vesicovaginal) or between the bowel and the skin (enterocutaneous).

G

Gastroenterologist: A medical specialist in treating disorders of the esophagus, stomach, bowel, and rectum.

Genomics: The study of gene expression patterns.

Grade: A pathologist term that defines how abnormal a cell is under the microscope.

Gynecological oncologist: A specialist in the treatment of cancer of the female reproductive system.

H

Hematogenous dissemination: A process of spreading by which cancer travels through the bloodstream.

Hydronephrosis: Abnormal enlargement of the kidney.

Hydroureteronephrosis: Abnormal enlargement of the kidney and the tube where urine flows, called the ureter.

I

Intraperitoneal: Into the abdomen.

Intraperitoneal port: A device surgically placed under the skin and into the abdomen that allows directed treatment into the abdomen.

Intubation: Process by which a person is placed on a breathing machine.

K

Krukenberg tumor: A cancer that has gone into the ovary from another place, usually starting in the stomach.

L

Laparoscopy: Camera-directed surgery done without creating a large incision in the abdomen.

Laparotomy: Surgery through a large incision in the abdomen.

Letrozole: An anti-estrogen medication that works by blocking your body from making estrogen out of your own naturally occurring proteins.

Leuprolide acetate: An anti-hormone that blocks release of estrogen and progesterone at the level of the brain.

Lymphatic channels: Vessels through which lymph fluid travels; part of the lymphatic system.

Lymphatic spread: Metastasis of cancer cells through the lymphatic system.

Lymphatic system: A network of lymphatic channels, lymph nodes, and organs, such as the spleen and the tonsils, that forms the major component of the immune system.

M

Menopause: Physical changes marking the end of a woman's fertile years, the most notable change being the cessation of menstrual cycles.

Menstruation: Vaginal bleeding due to endometrial shedding following ovulation when the egg is not fertilized.

Metastases: Tumor that has spread to distant places in the body.

Metastatic: Adjective used to describe a tumor that has spread.

Mitosis: Process of cells dividing.

Mixed mesodermal tumors: Tumors of dual origin with one part consisting of carcinomas and the other part consisting of sarcoma, hence their other designation as a carcinosarcoma.

Moderately differentiated: A pathologist's term to describe cellular changes of a cancer cell; cells that do not resemble their normal appearance but are still recognizable as related to their normal counterparts.

Multicompartmental: Multiple spaces, used to describe a finding seen in complex cysts on imaging studies, like ultrasounds.

Mutations: Genetic changes in DNA; mutations are not always harmful but sometimes can be associated with cancer development.

N

Nasogastric (NG) tube: A tube placed temporarily through the nose (naso) into the stomach (gastric) to help relieve continuous vomiting caused by a bowel obstruction.

Neoadjuvant treatment: Treatment given before surgery.

O

Omental cake: Tumor involvement of the omentum that results in the formation of a large mass.

Omentum: Fatty apron that drapes from the stomach and colon.

Optimal debulking: Surgical result if residual tumor is less than 1cm in diameter at the end of surgery.

Ovulation: Process of egg release from the ovary.

P

Palliation: To provide relief of pain. Adj.: palliative.

Papilla: Budding formations on structures, seen on ultrasound or other imaging.

Paracentesis: The process of removing ascites.

Pathological remission: The finding of no residual cancer at the end of primary treatment for cancer; only diagnosed in a second surgical procedure.

Patient-controlled analgesia (PCA): A method of providing pain medication through the vein that allows direct control over the amount required to make one comfortable.

Percutaneous endoscopic gastrostomy (PEG): A tube placed by a gastroenterologist that is inserted through your skin (percutaneous) and into your stomach using a flexible tube containing a camera (endoscopic). A hole is made in the stomach (gastrotomy) and the tube is fixed from the stomach and exits the skin. The purpose is to allow continuous drainage of bowel contents in a woman with terminal cancer who has an intractable bowel obstruction.

Perforation: Rupture of the wall of the bowel.

Performance status: A numerical description of how a person is doing in her normal day-to-day life and whether her cancer is impacting her ability to live normally.

Peritoneal carcinomatosis: Involvement of the omentum or bowels with cancer, usually the size of "rice granules" or tumor nodules.

Peritoneal cavity: The abdominal space.

Peritoneal seeding: The process of cancer spreading to involve the peritoneal surface.

Peritoneovenous shunt: Device that allows drainage of ascites from the peritoneum directly back into the bloodstream.

Peritoneum: The lining of the peritoneal cavity.

Pleural effusion: Fluid build-up around the lungs.

Pleurodesis: Process performed to prevent further build-up of fluid around the lung.

Poorly differentiated: A pathologist's term to describe cellular changes of a cancer cell; this describes cells that bear no resemblance to their normal counterparts.

Primary peritoneal cancer: Cancer that arises from the lining of the gut, or the peritoneum. This cancer behaves similarly to ovarian cancer and is treated much in the same way.

Prognosis: An estimate of the outlook following the diagnosis of a disease such as cancer.

Prophylactic oophorectomy: Removal of a woman's ovaries in an attempt to reduce or remove a risk for ovarian cancer in the future.

Proteomics: The study of protein profiles.

Pulmonary fibrosis: Scarring of the lung tissue, which may or may not be reversible.

R

Regeneration: To grow back.

Renin: A hormone released by the kidney normally that is important in maintaining hydration.

Reservoir: A receptacle that holds fluid.

S

Second-line chemotherapy: Chemotherapy given during recurrence.

Sensory neuropathy: Numbness and tingling, usually involving the hands and feet.

Septations: Thin membranes or walls dividing an area into multiple chambers. Often used to describe complex cysts seen on ultrasound.

Serological relapse: Diagnosis of recurrence solely based on an elevation of a tumor marker without evidence of recurrence by radiology tests.

Sporadic: Isolated; to occur without a pattern.

Suboptimal debulking: Residual disease greater than 1 cm in diameter upon completion of surgery.

Surgical staging: Procedure of determining the extent of cancer present.

T

T-cells: Immune cells that primarily fight viruses. They are being used in clinical trials of immunotherapy for ovarian and other cancers.

Theca-lutein cysts: Functional cysts that occur in the ovary due to the cyclic changes of hormones during a woman's period.

Thoracentesis: Procedure of draining a pleural effusion.

Thoracic surgeon: A surgeon who has completed extra training in the surgical management of diseases involving the chest and its organs.

Torsion: Act of twisting or turning in on itself (ovarian torsion, for example).

Total hysterectomy: Surgical excision of the uterus and cervix.

Total parenteral nutrition (TPN): Nutrition that is given by vein.

Treatment-free interval: The time between the end of one chemotherapy regimen and initiation of a subsequent therapy for recurrent disease.

Treatment holiday: A break in treatment that allows the body time to recover from toxicity.

True negative rate: The proportion of patients who have a negative test result and who do not have the disease.

True positive rate: The proportion of patients who have a positive test result and who do have the disease.

Tumor: A mass of cells that grow abnormally.

U

Undifferentiated: A pathologist's term to describe cellular changes of a cancer cell; this describes cells that bear no resemblance at all to normal cells.

Ureter: The anatomical structure that enables us to get rid of urine. It connects the kidney to the bladder.

V

Vaccine: A preparation that is given to induce immunity to a disease or condition.

W

Well-differentiated: A pathologist's term to describe cellular changes of a cancer cell; this describes cells that meet the criteria for cancer but still maintain a resemblance to normal cells.

Index